Domiciliary Palliative Care

A Handbook for Family Doctors and Community Nurses

Oxford General Practice Series ● 27

DEREK DOYLE, OBE, FRCSEd, FROPEd, FRCGP
Medical Director
St Columba's Hospice, Edinburgh

With a foreword by Dr Alastair G. Donald

OXFORD NEW YORK TOKYO
OXFORD UNIVERSITY PRESS
1994

Oxford University Press, Walton Street, Oxford OX2 6DP
Oxford   New York
Athens   Auckland   Bangkok   Bombay
Calcutta   Cape Town   Dar es Salaam   Delhi
Florence   Hong Kong   Istanbul   Karachi
Kuala Lumpur   Madras   Madrid   Melbourne
Mexico City   Nairobi   Paris   Singapore
Taipei   Tokyo   Toronto
and associated companies in
Berlin   Ibadan

Oxford is a trade mark of Oxford University Press

Published in the United States
by Oxford University Press Inc., New York

A catalogue record for this book is available from the British Library

Library of Congress Cataloging in Publication Data
Doyle, Derek.
Domiciliary palliative care : a guide for the primary care team /
Derek Doyle ; with a foreword by Alistair G. Donald.
(Oxford medical publications) (Oxford general practice series ; 27)
Includes bibliographical references.
1. Terminal care.   2. Palliative treatment.   3. Home care services.
I. Title.   II. Series.   III. Series : Oxford general practice series ; no. 27.
[DNLM: 1. Palliative Treatment—methods.   2. Home Care Services.
3. Primary Health Care.   W1 OX55 no. 27 1994 / WB 310 D754da 1994]
R726.8.D6799   1994   362.1'75—dc20   94-30956
ISBN 0 19 262489 X (Pbk)

Set by Advance Typesetting Ltd, Oxfordshire
Printed in Great Britain by
Redwood Books, Trowbridge, Wilts

Foreword

Dr Alastair G. Donald CBE, MA, FRCPE, FRCGP
President of the Royal College of General Practitioners

It is a particular pleasure to introduce and welcome this handbook for family doctors and community nurses on the theme of domiciliary palliative care. Like so many of my colleagues in general practice, I owe a great personal debt to the author, Derek Doyle, for the role he has played in developing the understanding and skills that have allowed the care of the dying patient to develop into a clinical discipline with its own educational content. I learned from him many things of a simple nature and others more technical. Above all I learned to understand the characteristics of pain, how to anticipate it and how to relieve it and thereby permit many patients to lead a meaningful life, in contact with friends and family, almost to the last moment. I learned, too, skills in manipulating the medicines at my command to relieve many of the discomforts experienced by the dying.

The discipline of palliative medicine has developed remarkably through the work of Derek Doyle and colleagues in the hospice movement, inheriting the tradition of Dame Cicely Saunders, and working in close collaboration with members of the primary health care team in the community as well as with specialist colleagues. Their work has gone a long way to conquer the fear of 'the last enemy'.

This book contains a wealth of information and advice on all aspects of palliative care with particular reference to its application in a community setting. Practical skills and knowledge are, however, blended with compassion and an awareness that there is a spiritual dimension to life. The book will, therefore, inform and inspire those who have the responsibility and the privilege of caring for patients afflicted with mortal disease. There was a time when domiciliary midwifery bonded general practitioners, midwives, and nurses to patients and their families. Today much of that bonding has been replaced by the care that we can offer to the dying and the rewards are equally great.

The motto of the Royal College of General Practitioners is 'Cum Scientia Caritas' meaning science blended with compassion and these words sum up the content of this book which I am delighted to commend.

Preface

It is said that most people would prefer to die at home. That may be so, but the fact remains that whilst 90 per cent of the last year is spent at home, fewer people are dying at home than ever before. The reasons for this are many and complex and beyond the scope of this book. Clearly, however, they are not all medical reasons, for there is ample evidence of excellent primary care in Britain and many other countries, with increasing numbers of vocationally trained doctors interested in good palliative care, community nurses equally committed to such care, and better resources than ever before to make it possible. Still the numbers who die at home continue to fall.

What is known is that the standard of palliative care varies greatly from district to district, practice to practice, and of course from country to country; that there are many references to deficiencies and failings which could, and should, be corrected and that there is now so much knowledge about every aspect of palliative care that no one can now plead ignorance.

The most common deficiencies reported in the literature relate to the quality of pain and symptom control, the planning of care, the response to emergencies, and the quality of cooperation and communication between the many professionals, and the patients and their relatives. All of these issues will be addressed in this text.

Whether or not the trend towards fewer home deaths will continue is not our concern here. Our concern is that, while patients are under the care of primary health care teams, they have the best care possible, and that the members of these teams may gain the knowledge, confidence, and deep professional satisfaction which can be such a feature of modern palliative care.

The days are long past when any doctor, specialist or generalist, need say, 'There is no more that I can do'. Today, there is the possibility of 'doing' and 'being' as compassionately and skilfully as at any other time in a patient's care. This book reaffirms the commitment of every member of a good primary care team faced with a patient coming to the end of a mortal illness − 'There is so much now we can all do!'.

Edinburgh   D.D.
May 1994

Contents

1 Pain palliation

The importance of pain and our ability to control it cannot be exaggerated. In cancer patients near the end of life, it is one of the most common symptoms, second only to asthenia and lethargy, and beyond doubt the most feared symptom. Even in other mortal illnesses not usually regarded by doctors as being associated with pain, it is nevertheless expected and feared by patients and carers. The fact that it is experienced by only 25 per cent of non-cancer patients, and by about 70 per cent with malignant disease, is not widely known by the general public. What they do know is that our ability to control it seems less than perfect. Almost everyone can cite examples of terrible suffering in family members or friends, facts borne out in many surveys and studies. Our patients have reason to dread it and we have good reason to ask how this poor record of care came about when we have such a range of analgesics at our disposal. The reasons are many and include:

(1) waiting for the patient to complain and then expecting him to describe the pain in graphic and helpful detail as he would *acute* pain. (Chronic pain is totally different from acute pain: it is less often reported, is usually described undramatically and almost apologetically, has a less well-defined starting point, no end point, little diagnostic value (except to define the precise cause of the pain rather than the primary pathology) and is without exception deeply distressing and depressing, rapidly destroying any quality of life.)

(2) the failure of the doctor or nurse to elicit precise details of *each* pain and to keep each other fully informed of all the patient describes and experiences. (Too often it is merely noted that 'the patient has pain' with no attempt to define and record the relevant details which are absolutely essential if it is to be treated specifically.);

(3) prescribing the right drug in the wrong dose or frequency or without the appropriate co-analgesics;

(4) withholding strong opioids because of the misplaced fears of addiction, tolerance, respiratory depression, or 'inevitable nausea and vomiting';

(5) failure to consider the use of radiotherapy, nerve blocks, hormones, cytotoxic chemotherapy, antibiotics, and neurosurgical procedures in the control of pain in malignant disease;

(6) failure to review regularly and frequently the patient's pattern of suffering, the development of new pains, and the regimen being used;

(7) failure to take into account the complex emotional, social, and spiritual factors present in every patient with far advanced illness;
(8) minimal experience in titrating drugs to match patients' needs—something seldom done in general practice except in diabetics.

THE PRINCIPLES OF PAIN CONTROL

Make an accurate diagnosis of *each* pain, remembering that most patients will have at least three or four different pains. They can be classified as:

(1) *pain due to the principal pathology* (e.g. cancer and its metastases, arthritides, inflammatory conditions, degenerative disease etc.) accounting for 65 per cent of pains;
(2) *pain due to the treatment* (e.g. post-operative, adhesions and their sequelae) accounting for 5 per cent of pains;
(3) *pain due to associated conditions* (e.g. pressure sores, oedema, constipation) accounting for a further 5 per cent;
(4) *pain due to unrelated pre-existing conditions* (e.g. osteoarthritis, rheumatoid arthritis, post-herpetic neuralgia) accounting for 25 per cent of pains.

Both doctor and nurse must discipline themselves never to ask merely, 'Have you any pain?' but rather to say, 'Do you have any pain anywhere? If so, I want you to describe each and every pain you have in as much detail as you possibly can'. Only then will they, for example, describe the sore mouth of candidiasis, the pain in each bone metastasis, the quite separate and different pain emanating in a stretching liver capsule, the discomfort of chronic constipation, the night cramp, and the vague but deeply distressing discomfort of neuropathic pain. All may coexist in the single patient, and each requires a different regimen and each calls for regular review.

On *each* subsequent visit to the patient, the doctor and nurse must invite the patient to report on *each* pain, in *each* site, and make whatever therapeutic changes are needed.

THE TYPES OF PAIN

Pharmacologically, it is possible to describe pain types in terms of opioid sensitivity, (i.e. opioid-sensitive, opioid-resistant, and opioid-partially sensitive), but this is not as helpful to us in domiciliary care as attempting to define pain by its cause and site.

1. *Bone pain* may be due to metastases, osteoporosis, collapse or fractures and Paget's disease.

(a) A fracture or collapse must be suspected when severe pain develops acutely in a well-defined area clearly identified by the patient.

(b) Osteoporosis or Paget's disease will probably have been suffered or suspected for some time before the terminal phase and confirmed radiologically and biochemically.

(c) Metastases, particularly in the patient known to have a malignancy, will be described as a dull ache over an area the size of a hand and then the patient will use the tip of a finger to demonstrate the site of exquisite pain and tenderness in a bone. The strong clinical suspicion of metastases will then be confirmed by a straight X-ray followed if needed by an isotope bone scan, together with estimation of alkaline phosphatase (and iso-enzymes), calcium, and albumin.

2. *Visceral pain* may be produced by tumour secondaries and in an organ such as liver, spleen, or kidney, the pain being produced by stretching of the capsule. It is described as a sickening, dull, deep-seated ache over the affected organ, made worse on palpation. It has to be remembered that the first site of hepatic pain is under the posterior right ribs, worse when the patient bends forward and eased by lying flat or on the right side. As the hepatomegaly increases, the pain is more apparent in the right axillary line and the patient cannot lie on the left side without increasing the discomfort. By the time hepatomegaly is palpable in the right hypochondrium, the pain is diffuse round the back, side and hypochondrium, and the patient can only find comfort when propped up on pillows, unable to lie flat or bend forward. Even then there may still not be gross derangement of the liver function tests.

3. *Nerve compression pain* is produced by external pressure on the nerve by the tumour or its secondaries and affected nodes. It is described as burning or stabbing, strictly confined to one or more adjacent dermatomes, the patient almost always using a single finger or his fingernail to demonstrate the fine line of its spread.

4. *Cerebral pain* due to cerebral oedema, the underlying primary or secondary tumour, or a focal metastasis in one of the cranial bones. With the former it is usually demonstrated by the patient holding his whole head in his hands, describing it as 'dull', 'oppressive', or 'like a vice', often present only in the morning and on straining. When due to a local cranial secondary, the patient always localizes it and prefers to keep his finger pressing on it to relieve the pain.

5. *Colic* is described in the classical way as intermittent, short-lived but building up in a crescendo and recurring at regular intervals.

6. *Muscular and arthritic pains*, no different from at any other time of life, are localized to the offending part and clearly relate to the use of a particular muscle group or joint.

7. *Neuropathic pain*, quite unlike all other pains, is caused principally by direct infiltration of a nerve by tumour or by diabetes mellitus. Many patients will state that this is an 'ache', a 'terrible discomfort' rather than a pain but its

recognition is vitally important because it will not respond to opioids but rather to other drugs to be detailed later. Because the nerve function is inevitably disturbed, there may be features of dysaesthesia or allodynia (pain produced by non-noxious stimulation). The doctor and nurse would be well advised always to ask, 'Do you have any area where it is not really pain but more a persistent ache—an area of numbness?'. Any patient who says he has discomfort or an ache in a numb area is not contradicting himself. He probably has neuropathic pain which merits skilled attention.

THE ANALGESIC LADDER

The World Health Organization analgesic ladder has been tested and validated in countless studies worldwide. It is effective. Why, then, do more doctors not follow it? Even when, as we shall describe, the specific measures for different pains are applicable, the analgesic ladder can still be the basis for good pain management (Fig. 1.1).

Step 1—non-opioids (for example, paracetamol): the patient is prescribed paracetamol and the dose is increased to the maximum recommended, tolerated dose and maintained at that so long as analgesia is satisfactory. When pain is not controlled, the doctor moves the patient to *Step 2*.

Step 2—weak opioids (such as codeine, coproxamol, cocodamol, codydramol, and dihydrocodeine): there is little, if anything, to choose between these different drugs and preparations. The patient is prescribed one of them and the dose

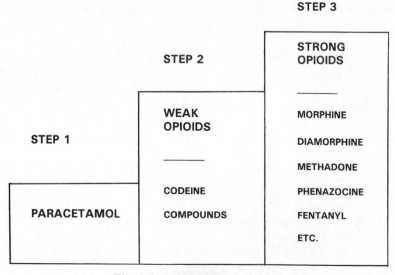

Fig. 1.1   WHO analgesic ladder.

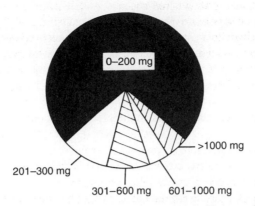

Fig. 1.2 1000 Patients with lung cancer oral morphine requirement/day.

is increased to the maximum recommended, tolerated dose and maintained there so long as analgesia is satisfactory. When pain control is lost, there is nothing to be gained by changing to another compound in this group and the doctor should move to *Step 3*.

Step 3—strong opioids (such as morphine, diamorphine, methadone, phenazo-cine, and fentanyl): starting with a morphine solution 5 milligram every 4 hours, the dose is titrated up until pain is controlled irrespective of how long is thought to be the patient's prognosis. Two things need to be remembered about strong opioids—'the younger the patient the higher the dose needed' and the dose depends on renal not hepatic function because renal insufficiency leads to accumulation of active metabolites.

STRONG OPIOID PREPARATIONS

1. Morphine solution should be the preparation of choice while establishing the required dose before any change is made to slow-release morphine preparations. A proprietary preparation may be used, or morphine sulphate in chloroform water (always made up to 10 ml dose). There is no merit whatsoever in using diamorphine solution.
2. Immediate-release morphine tablets are preferable for those who dislike the unpalatability of the solution but some patients will dislike having to take many tablets or be upset by the frequent changes in prescription and number of tablets while titration is taking place.
3. Slow-release morphine (SRM—for example, MST Continus) now comes in tablet and dispersable form in a range of strengths, each designed to main-tain a therapeutic plasma level for 12 hours. It is an excellent preparation for use when the opioid requirement has been defined but, as it takes up to

4 hours to achieve the desired plasma level, cannot be used 'as required' for incident or breakthrough pain.

4. Morphine suppositories are available in a range of strengths and useful for the occasional patient unable/unwilling to take oral medication but they need to be used 4–6 hourly in the same dose as the oral medication they are replacing. With increasing use of syringe-drivers, they are now seldom needed.

5. Diamorphine—because of its excellent solubility, this, and not morphine, is the preferred drug for injections and therefore for use via a syringe-driver. It has no other benefits over morphine.

6. Fentanyl, long used by anaesthetists, is now to become available in the UK as a transdermal patch, as it has been for some time in North America. This only needs to be replaced every 72 hours, a considerable boon to the patient who need not then take oral or injected opioids. Like MST, it is expensive.

7. Methadone is available in tablet, syrup, and injection form. This drug is a useful strong opioid but it has a long half-life, unpredictable sedation, and depression of respiration, and no advantages over morphine and diamorphine.

8. Dextramoramide (Palfium) is available in tablet form (which can be sucked sublingually) and as a suppository. This drug is three times as potent as oral

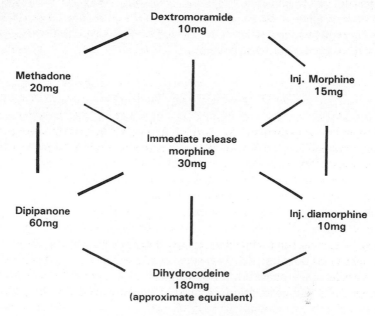

Fig. 1.3   Analgesic equivalents.

Table 1.1 *Duration of effectiveness of principal opioids used in palliative care*

Drug	Duration
Dextromoramide	2 hours
Immediate-release morphine	4 hours
Co-codeine preparations ⎫	
Dipipanone ⎬	6 hours
Phenazocine ⎭	
Methadone	8 hours
Slow-release morphine (MST)	12 hours
Fentanyl TTS	72 hours

morphine but the plasma level is maintained for no more than 2 hours, making it useful for 'incident' pain or to provide analgesia during a painful procedure but *never* for maintenance opioid therapy. Tolerance can develop rapidly. It is a valuable drug in domiciliary care to help the community nurse do painful dressings or catheter care because of its rapid onset of action, short period of action, and no longterm sedation.

9. Phenazocine (Narphen) is a little-used opioid agonist. It has 4—5 times the potency of oral morphine and can be given every six hours. Its sedative effect varies considerably, as does its respiratory depressant potential, and in all other respects it has no advantage over morphine or diamorphine. It is useful in domiciliary care for the occasional patient who is averse to taking morphine and requires a morphine equivalent of up to 100 milligram per day.

10. Dipipanone (Diconal) is only available in the UK combined with cyclizine. It is half the potency of oral morphine, needs to be given every six hours and is useful only when a morphine equivalent of up to 40 milligram a day is required. For most patients it is preferable when moving from a weak opioid to a strong opioid to go straight to morphine solution, bypassing this drug.

Opioids by injection

The drug of choice is diamorphine because of its solubility. It may be given by intermittent injection every 4 hours where oral preparations are inappropriate for any reason and the dose requirement is still being defined. When the daily requirement has been ascertained, it is then useful to transfer the patient to a syringe-driver. Alternatively, it may be given by syringe-driver, with the syringe loaded with the 24-hour requirement, changed daily by the community nurse. To the diamorphine may be added one (and preferably no more) of the drugs below:

- midazolam
- hyoscine hydrobromide
- hyoscine butylbromide
- chlorpromazine

- methotrimeprazine
- promazine
- prochlorperazine

- haloperidol
- droperidol
- dexamethasone ⎫ equally effective
       and ⎬
- betamethasone ⎭ and stable
- metoclopramide
- cyclizine (produces a white precipitate)

Use of a syringe-driver (see Appendix 1 and Fig. 1.4(a) and (b))

The following points should be noted:

1. The preferred sites are the abdominal wall, the anterior chest wall in the anterior axillary line, and over the deltoid insertion.
2. Provided the site remains healthy, it need not be changed more often than every 4 days, with a new giving set every 7−10 days.
3. A sterile inflammatory reaction (looking exactly like an injection abscess) occurs in about 10 per cent of cases, usually related to the amount of opioid

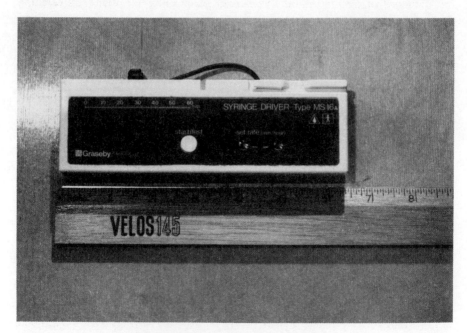

Fig. 1.4 (a)   Syringe-driver and ruler.

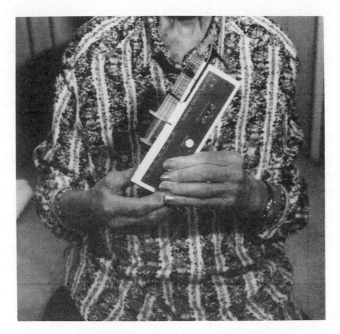

Fig. 1.4 (b)   Syringe-driver.

used or the added cyclizine. It is sometimes possible to prevent this occurrence if hyaluronidase (Hyalase), 1500 IU, is added to the syringe-driver or
separately injected into the infusion site.
4. The infusion must always be subcutaneous, never intramuscular. Clearly it
may be inappropriate and impracticable in a patient emaciated with malignant
cachexia.

MANAGING SPECIFIC PAINS

The general principles of pain management and the use of opioids have been
described. They apply whatever the cause and site of pain. One of the secrets
of good palliative care pain control in these patients is the defining of specific
pains and their *specific* treatment, rather than prescribing morphine and using
it like a fire blanket without any thought as to what is producing the pain.

Bone metastases

Any patient with malignant disease complaining of bone pain must be regarded
as having metastases until proved otherwise. The treatment will be as follows.

Palliative radiotherapy

This may be given in a single or divided fractions, remembering that side-effects of such treatment are usually no more than slight nausea and tiredness, but benefit is not seen for at least two weeks in most patients, occasionally earlier in patients with myeloma. An irradiated site cannot usually be re-irradiated but it is important for the family doctor to know exactly the site irradiated in case new pain is found to be outside that field. The sooner a patient suspected of having bone metastases is investigated and referred directly to the radiotherapist, the better.

Non-steroidal anti-inflammatory drugs (NSAIDs)

These exert their prostaglandin biosynthetase inhibitory effect because of the PGE_2 released by bone metastases. Provided there are no major contra-indications to their use, they should be commenced as soon as the diagnosis is suspected. There is little to choose between the many available drugs, the choice usually being between:

- diclofenac
- piroxicam
- flurbiprofen

- naproxen
- indomethacin
- benorylate.

The deciding factors are patient compliance, drug formulation and convenience of use, and the frequency the preparation must be taken. Diclofenac and flurbiprofen must be taken three times a day orally, naproxen twice a day, and piroxicam daily because of its long half-life and accumulation. Benorylate is useful when others are contraindicated because of dyspepsia. There is no convincing evidence that H_2 antagonists should be given concurrently.

Opioids

These are given as described above, always remembering that after several weeks when radiotherapy response shows, the opioid may be reduced. This is a timely reminder that the physiological antagonist of the opioid is pain. When pain is relieved (as by radiotherapy or a nerve block) the patient may then have more opioid in him than he needs and will then—for the first time—show such adverse effects as sedation, depression of respiration, and pinpoint pupils. He now needs less opioid. So long as a patient has any pain, there is no need to be on the alert for these signs.

This regimen will cope satisfactorily with most bone metastases. If not, usually advised by an oncologist or palliative medicine specialist, the patient may need a bisphosphonate (as for hypercalcaemia), salmon calcitonin, strontium, or an intraosseous injection of local anaesthetic, steroid, and/or phenol.

Visceral pain

This can be relieved with opioids as described (liver dysfunction is not a contraindication) or with steroids, for example, dexamethasone 4 milligram to 8 milligram early in the day in divided doses, reducing when pain lessens. The patient in whom it is inadvisable to give oral steroids can be given IM methylprednisolone (Depo-Medrone) 40 milligram twice-weekly at home.

Nerve compression pain

1. Steroids can be used to reduce perineural oedema. Dexamethasone is preferable to prednisolone because fewer tablets are needed. Usually adequate is 8 milligram per day reducing by 2 milligram per day every 2 or 3 days, as always taken as early in the day as possible. Occasionally it is necessary to continue with a maintenance dose of 2 milligram for a few weeks. The benefit is usually apparent within 48 hours.
2. Opioids can be used as described, a relatively low dose often being sufficient.
3. Nerve blocks may have a place if the pain is in dermatomes readily accessible for blockade. This is a modality seldom needed.

Nerve compression pain must be distinguished from neuropathic pain— different in all its characteristics and the drugs found effective.

Colic

With the possible exception of colic caused by subacute intestinal obstruction (so seldom amenable to surgery in patients with advanced cancer), colic is usually due to treatable if not reversible conditions such as:

- biliary colic (often associated with cholangitis)
- renal colic (due to calculi or clots)
- urinary tract infection, constipation, dysmenorrhoea.

Management therefore starts with defining, then treating, the underlying condition so far as is possible. The most useful anti-spasmodics in these patients are:

- prostaglandin biosynthetase inhibitors such as diclofenac
- mebeverine 135 milligram three times a day
- hyoscine butylbromide (Buscopan) by tablet or injection. It is useful to remember that this preparation can be given by syringe-driver, miscible with diamorphine, in a dose of 20–120 milligram over 24 hours.

It should be noted that opioid agonists such as morphine and diamorphine can actually make colic worse and that there is no place in palliative care for pethidine.

Skin hyperaesthesia (allodynia):

Allodynia is pain produced by non-noxious stimulants. The patient does not like light touch, or the irritating effect of tight clothing or heavy bedding. In palliative care it is reported by patients with:

- cerebro-vascular accidents
- small cell bronchogenic carcinoma
- reticuloses
- melanomatosis.

The management requires skilled nursing, skin cooling, generous application of talcum powder, loose clothing, lightweight bedding, and a bed cradle. Useful drugs worth trying are:

- H_2 antagonists such as cimetidine and ranitidine in the standard dose
- β-blockers (provided there are no contra-indications) such as propanolol 10 milligram three times a day
- salicylates or preparations combining salicylates and opioids (Aspav).

Neuropathic pain

Traditionally this pain, almost always opioid-resistant and usually described as an aching discomfort in a numb area, has two presentations.

The more common presentation is as a persistent, dull, gnawing ache, diffuse over a wide area, for example over a shoulder and upper arm, or a buttock, hip, and posterior thigh. Treatment for this type is amitriptyline, starting with 25 milligram nightly for 3 or 4 nights, then increased to 50 milligram for another 3 or 4 days, and finally to a maintenance dose of 75 milligram nightly. Benefit begins to show after 7−10 days and seldom will a higher dose be needed. If, for some reason, amitriptyline is unacceptable, other tricyclics may be used, for example, imipramine early in the day or nortriptyline at night. Neither the tetracyclics nor the newer families of antidepressants have any place in the management of neuropathic pain.

The less common presentation, but one which occasionally occurs in the group just described, is a momentary, intense, hot, stabbing pain in the affected area — 'like an electric shock'. This requires different drugs, such as sodium valproate 500 milligram three times a day or phenytoin 300 milligram daily or carbamazepine, slowly increased as necessary from 200 milligram daily to its maximum recommended dose of 1600 milligram daily, always on the alert for its serious adverse effects. Experience with many patients suffering this pain suggests that carbamazepine, whilst excellent for trigeminal neuralgia and some atypical facial pains, has less effect on neuropathic pain below the neck.

More recently, good results have been obtained with the cardiac cell membrane stabilizing drugs mexiletine (200−900 milligram per day) and flecainide.

It is not recommended that they should be commenced by the family doctor but rather started and monitored in a hospital or palliative care unit under the supervision of a consultant. Good results in lumbosacral plexopathy have been reported with subcutaneous ketamine 60–300 milligram/24 hours preferably given via a syringe-driver. Diabetic neuropathy has responded to paroxetine.

Muscular and arthritic pains are treated in exactly the same way at the end of life as at any other time and need no description here.

Incident pain ('breakthrough pain')

No matter how well controlled a patient's pain, there will be times when severe pain suddenly occurs, alarming the patient and carers, and demanding skilled attention by the family doctor. It is important to ascertain why this is happening.

1. Is it occurring so frequently and regularly as to suggest that the regular opioid dose should be increased? If this is the case, the doctor should increase the dose and not the frequency of administration. For example, if a patient on 10 milligram morphine solution reports pain frequently occurring about 30 minutes before his next dose is due, he should be changed to 15 milligram doses and not advised to take another dose whenever he feels pain. Otherwise, the routine will be out of control and the carers perplexed about how much it is safe for the patient to take.
2. Is it an infrequent event? In this case, he can be given 1/6 th of the total opioid intake on these occasions (i.e. the dose being taken every 4 hours by mouth, or 1/6 th of the diamorphine in the syringe-driver, or 1/6 th of the daily MST given not as MST but as immediate-release morphine).
3. Is it only during painful procedures? This is the indication for dextromoramide as already described or for Entonox if it can be obtained.

It cannot be stated strongly enough that each 'new' pain must be investigated and treated appropriately. It is not an indication for automatic increase in the opioid dose.

Coanalgesics

These are nonanalgesics which, combined with the analgesics described, can help to relieve pain. Examples already given include steroids, antidepressants and anticonvulsants. Others are:

(1) antibiotics and antifungals to relieve inflammatory reactions such as cellulitis, urinary tract infection (UTI), candidiasis;
(2) chemotherapeutic agents to reduce tumour or nodal bulk, stretching organ capsules, pressure on nerve plexuses;
(3) muscle relaxants such as diazepam and baclofen.

Other treatment options

Palliative radiotherapy

This has already been mentioned (see p. 10). In addition to its use in bone metastases, it is invaluable for spinal cord compression (SCC), superior vena caval obstruction (SVCO), haemoptysis, and to reduce tumour bulk particularly in the pelvis, retroperitoneal space, cranium, and porta-hepatis.

Transcutaneous electrical nerve stimulation (TENS)

Physiotherapists usually have more experience with TENS than most family doctors but advice can also be obtained from specialists in the pain clinic or palliative care unit (see Fig. 1.5(a) and (b)). The principal uses are in post-herpetic neuralgia and in soft tissue conditions but, in skilled and experienced hands, they can be used as adjuvants in patients with advanced cancer for many back and thoracic cage syndromes, perineal pain, and some neuropathic syndromes (see Appendix 2 and Fig. 1.6).

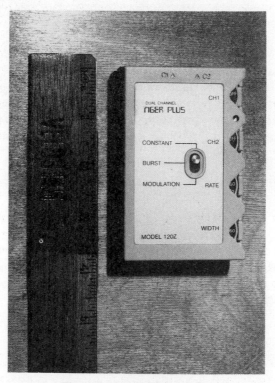

Fig. 1.5 (a)   TENS and ruler.

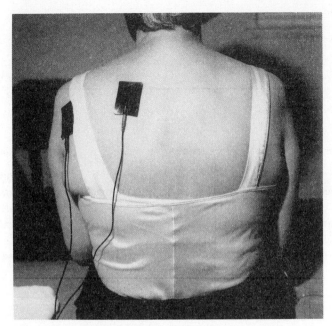

Fig. 1.5 (b) TENS in use.

Orthopaedic procedures

It is increasingly being recognized that the orthopaedic surgeon has an important role not only in fixation of pathological fractures and hip replacements, but in prophylactic procedures to stabilize the vertebral column and long bones before a fracture occurs. This, in itself, can reduce pain and the need for high-dose opioids.

Neurolytic procedures ('nerve blocks')

Whereas only a few years ago upwards of 20 per cent of patients suffering pain from advanced cancer were considered candidates for such procedures, that figure has now fallen to less than 5 per cent and in many centres they are not used at all. The reasons are our increasing knowledge of, and skills in using, the opioids and coanalgesics, the recognition that neurolytic procedures do not produce permanent relief from pain, and that their repetition is not without difficulties. Having said that, they have their uses.

Coelic plexus block for the pain of carcinoma of pancreas (L1) The earlier it is done the better. It requires 24–72 hours in hospital, the patient is awake during the procedure, and good results can be expected in about 75 per cent of cases. There may follow hypotension and diarrhoea.

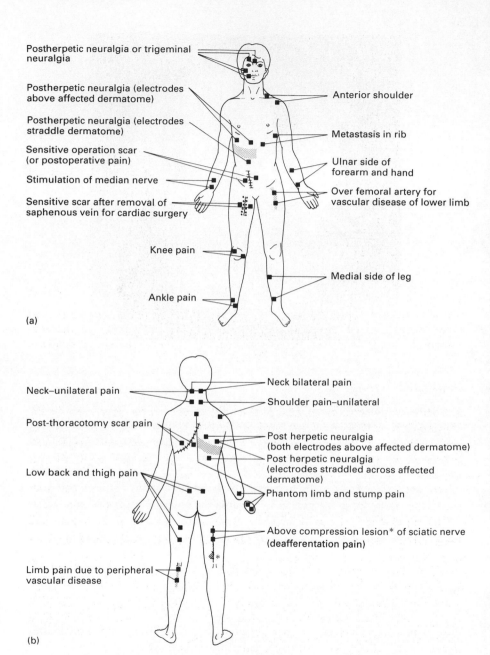

Postherpetic neuralgia or trigeminal neuralgia

Postherpetic neuralgia (electrodes above affected dermatome)

Postherpetic neuralgia (electrodes straddle dermatome)

Sensitive operation scar (or postoperative pain)

Stimulation of median nerve

Sensitive scar after removal of saphenous vein for cardiac surgery

Anterior shoulder

Metastasis in rib

Ulnar side of forearm and hand

Over femoral artery for vascular disease of lower limb

Knee pain

Ankle pain

Medial side of leg

(a)

Neck–unilateral pain

Post-thoracotomy scar pain

Low back and thigh pain

Limb pain due to peripheral vascular disease

Neck bilateral pain

Shoulder pain–unilateral

Post herpetic neuralgia (both electrodes above affected dermatome)

Post herpetic neuralgia (electrodes straddled across affected dermatome)

Phantom limb and stump pain

Above compression lesion* of sciatic nerve (deafferentation pain)

(b)

Fig. 1.6 Drawing of electrode positions commonly used for TENS. (a) Anterior aspect; (b) posterior aspect. Reproduced with permission from the *Oxford Textbook of Palliative Medicine*.

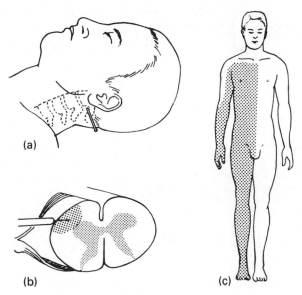

Fig. 1.7 (a) Site of percutaneous cordotomy. (b) Lesion produced by percutaneous C1–2 cordotomy. (c) Extent of analgesia produced by left C1–C2 percutaneous cordotomy. Reproduced with permission from the *Oxford Textbook of Palliative Medicine*.

Percutaneous cordotomy (PCC) This is probably more correctly a neuro-surgical procedure because it is often done by neurosurgeons in the UK but in some centres it is done by anaesthetists in a pain clinic. Originally employed principally for unilateral leg pain, it is now being used with good results for any unilateral pain, especially lumbro-sacral or brachial plexopathy. It is done with the patient conscious and able to cooperate, lying very still for at least one hour whilst the doctor passes a needle in towards the anterior spino-thalamic tracts on the opposite side, through the neck. Results are excellent if the patient will accept the degree of hypoaesthesia or dysaesthesia which result (see Fig. 1.7).

Other examples These include caudal blocks using steroids (and phenol if sphincter control has already been lost) for the relief of perineal pain; para-vertebral blocks for intrathoracic pain and that from a rapidly stretching liver capsule; intrathecal, epidural, and intercostal blocks, which are now done very infrequently but which show good results with subperiosteal and intraosseous injections in patients with recurrent pain in irradiated areas.

Neurosurgical

Procedures include PCC, open cordotomy, open rhizotomy, myelotomy, and stereotactic thalamotomy. It is important to reiterate that, useful as these procedures are, the average family doctor will practice for 20 years or more without encountering a patient who needs any of them.

QUESTIONS TO ASK

When the patient continues to report pain (or new pains develop), the doctor should ask the following questions:

1. Has the pain, or pains, been correctly diagnosed?
2. Are the correct drugs being used, in the right dose, at the right intervals?
3. Is the patient taking the drugs *exactly* as prescribed?
4. Is it a new pain and, if so, what is causing it?
5. Are there other influencing factors not being addressed — emotional, social, or spiritual?
6. Is there an underlying personality disorder leading to manipulative, attention-seeking behaviour?

When 'opioid-sensitive' pain fails to respond to opioids:

1. Is it an opioid-sensitive pain or only partially sensitive, e.g. bone pain, visceral pain, nerve compression?
2. Is the dose high enough, particularly in young patients ('the younger the patient the higher the dose')?
3. Is it a new pain, e.g. a pathological fracture, a distended bladder, or a loaded colon?
4. Is it neuropathic pain which is unlikely ever to respond to opioids?

THE ROLE OF THE PRIMARY CARE TEAM IN PAIN CONTROL

Some might deny it but it is almost impossible to achieve the level of pain control every patient deserves if family doctor and community nurse do not work together as an integrated team.

The doctor alone is able to prescribe but he can only do so effectively if each pain is identified accurately, and if the effect of the medication is monitored skilfully by himself and the nurse, taking into account the reports of the patient and family carers. This requires that the doctor and the nurse meet regularly to review:

- their care
- each pain and its control
- medication and the patient's cooperation.

It is important to be on the alert for new pains or changing descriptions of pain, to monitor adverse reactions, and to keep precise records of each pain, the treatment, and the treatment goals.

Some find Pain Assessment Charts useful (Appendix 5). They are not essential but do remind us of the subjective nature of pain, patterns we might not otherwise notice, the response or otherwise to medication and — probably more important than anything else — our commitment to good pain control, something still infrequently achieved.

2 Symptom palliation

THE PRINCIPLES

The following points are worth noting.

1. There may be several symptoms at any one time due both to the primary illness and to its complications. For example, a cancer patient may have symptoms resulting from the primary lesion and from multiple metastases in several organs or tissues, each of which may produce different symptoms. The fungating carcinoma of breast will produce its own problems but the same patient may have pain from bone metastases, discomfort from constipation, a sore mouth as a result of candidiasis, diplopia from cerebral metastases, and the many symptoms of hypercalcaemia. The cardiac patient may have myocardial ischaemic pain, dyspnoea, lethargy, and the discomfort of bed sores from having to sit for so long.

2. Treatment of the underlying or primary condition may be useful but will not necessarily alleviate the many other symptoms each of which must be identified.

3. Patients rarely want palliative treatment for each and every symptom simultaneously but they do have a right to hope that the professionals will be able to manage each one as and when they are troublesome. For example, most patients will put pain relief at the top of their list of priorities and be happy if something can be done to relieve their constipation, yet not expect concurrent attention to anorexia, sore mouth, lethargy, or their psychosocial problems until the pain and constipation have been relieved.

4. Such patients have many more problems than they admit. In fact they usually report as symptoms about only 50 per cent of their problems and these are not necessarily those which most worry them. They are more usually the symptoms about which they have been most frequently asked, i.e. those which most interest the doctor or nurse. The previously unreported problems (not 'symptoms' since they are not expressed) are not mentioned, unless the patient is encouraged to speak of them. He fears that the problems may be regarded as trivial, taking up too much of the doctor's precious time! 'Not reported' means only that — 'not reported' — and not that problems do not exist or are not worrying the patient.

5. Behind most symptoms lie unspoken fears which may never be expressed unless the doctor or nurse encourages the patient to speak of these fears. To the inexperienced or insensitive doctor, these fears may appear irrational or unfounded. They are not so to the patient whose life is coming to an end.

Every such fear must be addressed. Some common concerns may illustrate these fears and misunderstandings. The patient, sweating copiously because of his advanced carcinoma, often fears he has an infectious or contagious disease, and may secretly wonder if he has tuberculosis (because he has seen grandparents die of this), or even if he has AIDS.

The person who wakens up disorientated after his sleep and who feels he is not remembering things so well may wonder if he is developing a mental illness, forgetting those many other times when he was well and had the same experience. The tiniest fleck of blood in sputum may not surprise or worry the doctor who knows the patient has a bronchogenic carcinoma, but the patient is very likely to be anxious, not about the diagnosis, but whether it is a foretaste of a fatal haemorrhage.

6. A deliberately vague, euphemistic explanation by the doctor, given with the kindest of intentions, may not help the patient as much as the simple, straight truth expressed in a caring, sensitive manner. Even more confusing and hurtful is a vague explanation when it appears to conflict with an explanation given by another professional colleague. This frequently happens in domiciliary care. Terminally ill patients describe how much safer they feel when given the truth. 'I wouldn't worry about that sweating', the doctor may say but the patient is not helped when another doctor or nurse comes in and says, 'I wonder if you have an infection somewhere?'. The nurse may try to reassure the patient with blood in his sputum and ask the doctor to visit and advise, but when his first words are: 'Now let's see where that little haemorrhage has come from', fears will not be reduced.

7. Symptoms, expressed or suffered in silence, change very frequently, often several times in a day. Each visit by each professional must be an occasion for every aspect of suffering to be ventilated and dealt with. Only one coughing bout or acute dyspnoeic attack is needed to unnerve the patient.

HOW SHOULD THE PROFESSIONALS BEHAVE?

1. Professionals must train themselves to ask about everything which troubles the patient, and not merely about what interests the doctor! How easy it is to go in and ask, 'How's the pain today?' when the patient has not had pain for days but is known to be anxious about newly-developed dyspnoea, nausea, pruritus, or insomnia. The simple solution is to ask as a routine two-part question. 'How are you today? Tell me about everything which has troubled you since I saw you.' It helps if the doctor or nurse adds, 'It doesn't matter how silly it sounds—if it's worrying or upsetting you, I want to hear about it'.

2. Ask the patient to prioritize symptoms. They will nearly always be able to do so: 'I've lost my appetite and can't enjoy anything, but what really worries

me is this feeling of nausea;' 'I'm weak and tired and can't sleep but what I'd like you to do is to explain this funny feeling I get down here.'

3. Ask direct questions! 'I can see you're not so well today and you look anxious. What's on your mind? What do you think is going on in there to make you so breathless/nauseated/itchy/sleepless?'. One can safely be even more direct or blunt with many patients, 'Are you lying there wondering if you're going to bleed and bleed? If you are, I can explain all this to you and then give you something to help it'.

   Here the family doctor is often ideally placed to help. He knows the family background and may have looked after relatives, and can say things like 'Are you wondering if you're going to develop the same problems your mother had?' or 'This is like that time you had a terrible cough a few years ago and look how we managed to beat that.'

4. Respect every symptom, never hinting that anything is trivial, because when you are dying, nothing is trivial. 'Go on, tell me about it—if it's troubling you in any way, I want to hear so that I can help.'

5. Keep accurate records of the symptoms reported at each visit, detailing those being explained or treated and others which should be asked about on subsequent visits. 'You mentioned hiccup last week but didn't want me to do anything for it. How is it now?'

6. Share every detail, every explanation, and every management plan with the other colleagues involved so that everyone works towards the same goal, with harmonious explanations and a visible unity of purpose.

7. Explain the basis of each symptom and the rationale and goal of all treatment, simply, accurately, and honestly. 'You are short of breath because of slight congestion, a gathering of fluid in your lung. This white tablet will get rid of it and you'll notice you will pass more water.'

ANOREXIA

Principal causes

- dry mouth (xerostomia), often drug-induced
- oral candidiasis (present in 75 per cent of these patients)
- chronic constipation
- nausea and vomiting
- uninteresting, unimaginative food (often in too large servings and offered only at standard meal times)
- odours in the environment
- anxiety but more commonly depressive state
- metabolic—hypercalcaemia, elevated liver function tests (LFTs), uraemia etc.

Management

1. Try to identify and remove the offending cause(s).

2. Offer small helpings of attractively served food at frequent intervals un-related to standard meal times, preferably on the smallest plates available.
3. Terminally ill patients often eat good breakfasts, small midday meals, and take little or nothing in the evening. They often like 'breakfast' food such as cereals or porridge, at any time of day or night, and rarely refuse ice cream, sorbet, yogurt, or cold custard, no matter how much they disliked them before their illness.

    Coloured food is more tempting than drab but tasty food, hence the need for ice cream dressing, parsley on fish, thin, colourful slices of peppers even though they will not eat them, kiwi fruit slices, sauces or gravy on potatoes.

    Be reluctant to offer 'invalid' food, no matter how nutritious and skilfully promoted. Be ever ready to encourage any bizarre fancy the patient has, for example a Chinese carry-out, porridge in the middle of the night, a lager at breakfast, or stout with added sugar.
4. Suggest a small alcoholic aperitif, preferably chilled.

Drugs When all the above have been tried, consider prescribing.

(a) steroids: prednisolone 15 milligram per day for first week; 10 milligram per day for second week; 5 milligram per day for third week then discon-tinuing because there is no evidence that more extended use maintains appetite. The dexamethasone equivalent would be 2 milligram, 1.5 milli-gram, and 1 milligram, always taken before 2 p.m.
(b) megestrol acetate (Megace) in a dose of not less than 160 milligram per day for at least one month, continued if appetite improves and weight gain is shown. Studies have suggested the optimum dose is 480 milligram per day, but few patients can take so many tablets on top of their other medication (and the price is prohibitive).

ANTIBIOTICS IN PALLIATIVE CARE

Antibiotics have a place in palliative care: the relief of suffering rather than the saving of a life. In a patient with only days of life left, an acute infection can indeed be 'the old man's friend'. In most others it brings added suffering in the form of fever, malaise, sweating, dehydration, confusion, constipation, the specific features of the system involved, and even more nursing problems. If some of this can be reduced, whilst realistically not trying to extend life, anti-biotics must be considered.

Simple guidelines may assist:

1. Where possible, try to get antibiotic sensitivities done on specimens but be prepared to prescribe an appropriate broad spectrum drug while awaiting results.

2. Prescribe the simplest regimen of an antibiotic, easy to swallow, with the fewest adverse effects. Very rarely, if ever, will injected antibiotics be needed.
3. Do not attempt to treat a UTI in a catheterized patient or in any organ invaded by malignancy.
4. Be alert for such adverse effects as nausea, diarrhoea, and candidiasis, which may be more troublesome than the original infection.

ANXIETY

Anxiety is a common problem with these patients, often showing itself as fear, worry, or apprehension and with such physical symptoms as agitation, palpitation, shortness of breath, and numbness. *It is vitally important to try to define the cause(s).*

Causes

1. The existence of the physical illness itself and its symptoms, particularly if everything has not been explained or conflicting explanations and advice have been given.
2. Symptoms have not been acknowledged and appropriately addressed.

Doctors often overlook the fact that each symptom can have an unexpressed significance for the patient which may never have occurred to the professionals, for example:

(a) Breathlessness—'Am I going to die fighting for breath?'
(b) Dysphagia—'Am I going to starve to death or choke trying to eat something?'
(c) Haemoptysis—'Am I going to bleed to death?'
(d) Pain—'Do they know how much I'm suffering or can they do nothing about it? Is this pain one they can't do anything about?'
(e) Confusion—'Am I going mad? Is this dementia? Will I be sent to a psychiatric hospital?'

Every single symptom may puzzle or be perceived as a further threat to these patients, but be expected and accepted by the professionals who *wrongly* continue to regard symptoms as pointers to a diagnosis. By this time in a patient's life, each symptom is a reflection of suffering—something to be relieved as speedily as possible.

3. The way the family deals with the illness, particularly if attempts are being made to care for the patient at home, where relatives may themselves be tense and anxious in their coping and unable to share their own feelings for

the patient or let the patient describe his feelings and fears (this is particularly the case when all concerned are bent on nurturing the 'conspiracy of silence');

4. Feature of the illness itself and any organic mental state, remembering hypoxia, renal or hepatic failure, cerebral metastases, anaemia, sepsis, poorly controlled pain, and the medications being given (clearly it is more appropriate to deal with the cause of hypoxia (if that is possible) or to give opioids and oxygen, than to prescribe anxiolytics; more appropriate to give brain irradiation for cerebral metastases or dexamethansone for cerebral oedema than to prescribe anxiolytics. Having said that, it should be remembered that dexamethasone, particularly if given late in the day, is a psychic stimulant capable of exciting the patient and grossly disturbing the sleep pattern, thus mimicking an agitated anxiety state, when in fact it is iatrogenic);

5. The patient being a longterm benzodiazepine user and failure to continue these drugs will exacerbate anxiety, restlessness, and agitation, (in the chronically ill, particularly the elderly, it may be several days after withdrawal of these drugs before the classical withdrawal features show);

6. A coping mechanism, coming to terms with dramatic life changes, a new environment, new carers, many new professionals to get to know and trust.

Management

It is essential to explore all of these causes before reaching for the prescription pad. The nurse and doctor sitting together and sharing their knowledge and insight should ask several questions.

Pre-prescription checklist

1. Has every symptom been identified, explained and, where appropriate, treated? (The dying patient rarely asks for 'something' for every symptom but needs to know that the doctor and nurse are aware of it and will deal with it when asked to do so.)

2. Has every fear been explored and all explanations by the different professionals been consistent?

3. Are any of the symptoms iatrogenic?

4. Is there a past history of anxiety or depression, benzodiazepine or alcohol dependence, or of psychiatric care?

Only after one has gone through this checklist can thought be given to appropriate medication (Table 2.1).

Where possible, prescribe a short-acting benzodiazepine such as lorazepam or oxazepam (both are metabolized by conjugation in the liver and therefore the safest drugs in patients with hepatic disorder). Should patients experience breakthrough or end-of-dose anxiety, they should be converted to longer-acting benzodiazepines such as diazepam or clonazepam. The latter drug is said to be

Table 2.1 *Anxiolytic drugs*

Generic name	Appropriate daily dosage range (milligram)	Route
Benzodiazepines		
Very short-acting		
midazolam	1.25−125 per 24 h	SC,IV
Short-acting		
lorazepam	0.5−2.0 three times daily	PO, SC, IM, IV
oxazepam	10−15 three times daily	PO
Intermediate-acting		
chlordiazepoxide	10−50 three times daily	PO
Long-acting		
diazepam	5−10 twice daily−four times daily	PO, IV, PR
clonazepam	0.5−2 twice daily−four times daily	PO
Non-benzodiazepine		
buspirone	5−20 three times daily	PO
Neurolytics		
haloperidol	0.5−5 every 2 hours−12 hours	PO, IV, SC, IM
chlorpromazine	10−50 as every 4 hours−12 hours	PO, IM, IV
methotrimeprazine	10−25 every 4 hours−8 hours	PO, SC, IM
thioridazine	10−75 three times daily−four times daily	PO
Antihistamine		
hydroxyzine	25−50 every four hours−6 hours	PO, SC, IV
Tricyclic antidepressants		
imipramine	10−150 bedtime	PO
amitriptyline	10−150 bedtime	PO

PO: by mouth; SC: subcutaneously; IM: intramuscularly; IV: intravenously.

particularly useful in patients with symptoms of depersonalization or derealization with seizure disorders, brain tumours, or mild organic mental disorders. Provided starting doses are low and the change to longer-acting benzodiazepines is made in small increments, there need be no fear of respiratory depression in these patients.

Neuroleptics such as thioridazine and haloperidol are useful when benzodiazepines fail to control symptoms and when psychotic symptoms such as delusions and hallucinations develop. The phenothiazines (chlorpromazine and methotrimeprazine) are useful when sedation is needed, but one must remember their anticholinergic effects and ability to produce hypotension. Possibly the best

Table 2.2 *Antidepressant drugs*

Generic name	Appropriate daily dosage range (mg)	Route
Tricyclic antidepressants		
amitriptyline	10–150	PO
doxepin	10–150	PO
imipramine	10–150	PO
nortriptyline	10–125	PO
clomipramine	10–150	PO
Second generation antidepressants		
fluoxetine	20–160	PO
trazodone	25–300	PO

neuroleptic for the agitated with dangerously impulsive behaviour is pericyazine 15–30 milligram daily, but safe in doses as high as 75–150 milligram daily for the most disturbed.

Buspirone, a non-benzodiazepine anxiolytic, is valuable in chronic anxiety or anxiety related to adjustment disorders but its onset of action is slow, on the order of 5–10 days. It will not block benzodiazepine withdrawal so one must be cautious when switching from a benzodiazepine to buspirone.

Tricyclic antidepressants are indicated when anxiety is a feature of depressive state but their sedative and anticholinergic effects must be remembered (see Table 2.2).

Benefit will always follow the use of appropriate listed drugs, but there may still be a place for relaxation techniques, music therapy, guided imagery, or hypnosis when employed by someone trained and experienced in their use in these patients. Sadly, there are some who would suggest them as first-line options, which they are not.

ASCITES

Malignancy is the cause of 10 per cent of all cases of ascites and 15–50 per cent of patients with malignant disease will develop the condition. Thirty per cent of women with ovarian carcinoma will have it at presentation and over 60 per cent by the time they die. It is associated with almost all the malignancies likely to be seen in family practice including the less common ones such as melanoma, mesothelioma, and myeloma.

Ascites can, of course, be a feature of non-malignant conditions which may eventually require palliative care, such as liver disease with portal hypertension, cardiac failure, nephrotic syndrome, and even tuberculosis. In all patients it must be regarded as serious but in two situations—ovarian carcinoma and lymphoma—it may well respond to active treatment of the underlying disease. In all others, the aim is comfort, sometimes (but not always) achieved with paracentesis.

Management

1. Therapeutic paracentesis is often required but it should be remembered that complete drainage in a patient with hepatomegaly and/or abdominal tumour masses may lead to an increase in pain when the 'cushioning effect' of the ascites has been removed.

   There is no way of predicting how often the procedure will be needed. If frequent, because of the inevitable upheaval for the domiciliary patient being readmitted to hospital or palliative care unit, it is sometimes preferable for a drain to be left in and the patient supplied with a bag as for an ileo-conduit. Should the family doctor feel this would be useful for, and acceptable to, the patient, he should so advise his hospital colleagues. Each time a paracentesis is performed, there is further reduction of the plasma albumin leading to the development of hypo-albuminaemic oedema. This is not a contraindication to paracentesis, but the patient and relatives should be aware of it because rarely would it be appropriate in these patients to replace the albumin.
2. Spironolactone 100–400 milligram per day can certainly slow down the reaccumulation of ascites but at the cost of some appetite loss and possibly gynaecomastia in men. Some would recommend frusemide (40–80 milligram) to initiate diuresis but care must be taken not to overdo diuresis, as one risks precipitating electrolyte imbalance, hepatic encephalopathy, or prerenal failure.
3. Peritoneo-venous shunts can be inserted, draining the fluid from the abdomen to the internal jugular vein. The procedure takes 30–60 minutes but results with malignant ascites have been disappointing, and there is a high operative mortality (30 per cent in liver disease and 15 per cent in malignant disease). The benefit is so short (only 3–4 weeks in patients with positive ascitic fluid cytology) that the treatment is rarely justified.

BLADDER PROBLEMS

Bladder pain is difficult to treat, yet incontinence a common problem for which much can be done, and haematuria occasionally responds to medication. Interestingly, although urinary incontinence is embarrassing for most patients and the cause of extra work for relatives, it is seldom a reason for a request for hospitalization; faecal incontinence is something few relatives ever feel they can cope with at home.

Incontinence

1. Urinary Tract Infection (UTI) is worth treating with an appropriate oral antibiotic, provided the patient does not have a catheter in or has bladder carcinoma. It is illogical to give an antibiotic in this case because the catheter or tumour acts as a foreign body and there is little chance of eradicating infection.
2. Structural changes in the bladder due to intra/extra vesical tumour or post-irradiation/post-operative fibrosis, often lead to incontinence and bypassing around urethral catheters. There is nothing which can be done except urinary diversion 'in a fit enough patient or the provision of a suprapubic catheter.
3. Retention with overflow, if not due to benign prostatic hypertrophy or a prostatic carcinoma, usually betokens spinal cord compression, described on p. 70. Retention follows the use of opioids in about 10 per cent of patients requiring them for pain.
4. The excessive sedation associated with hypnotics and opioids must be remembered.

Urinary retention

1. Urinary retention may be induced by anticholinergic drugs, tricyclic antidepressants, and opioids.
2. Neurological causes such as spinal cord compression, tumour infiltration, or damage of the sacral plexuses should be considered.
3. Faecal impaction is much more common than most people realize and must be investigated in all cases no matter how vehemently the patient protests he is not constipated.
4. Prostatic obstruction, from whatever cause, will in these patients necessitate a permanent indwelling catheter.

Dysuria and strangury

1. Infection can be treated, catheter inserted, and lavage done regularly to remove clot and debris.
2. Generalized bladder pain may be relieved with prostaglandin inhibitors such as flurbiprofen (100 milligram three times a day), naproxen (500 milligram three times a day), or diclofenac (50 milligram three times a day); more usually it will be necessary to institute longterm opioid therapy.
3. Strangury is difficult and disappointing to treat. Occasionally propantheline (15 milligram four times a day) will help, or hyoscine butylbromide (20−120 milligram per day orally or via a syringe-driver); or, as a last resort, a coeliac plexus block.

Haematuria

Here we are speaking of haematuria of known origin, where specific treatment has been given to the carcinoma of kidney or bladder.

1. Ethamsylate (500 milligram four times a day) may reduce capillary bleeding and be effective within 3 or 4 days.
2. Silver nitrate bladder instillation (in the catheterized patient) involves a daily instillation of 50–100 ml of 1:10 000 silver nitrate, instilled into the bladder with the catheter clamped, and left in the bladder for as long as the patient can tolerate it (not exceeding 30 minutes), after which the clamp is removed and free drainage resumed. This is done for 5–7 days.
3. Alum solution 1 per cent instillation is an alternative to silver nitrate, 100 ml being instilled daily in the same routine as for silver nitrate.

Bladder lavage

Chlorhexidine 1:5000 used daily is the preferable solution for infection and weekly for maintenance. For debris, and clot removal, daily saline lavage is adequate. Noxythiolin, expensive but useful for infection and as a modest haemostatic, must be used as a week's course, but alternatives are 0.5 per cent of acetic or citric acid as the first line treatment.

It cannot be overstressed that catheterization is a safe and useful procedure in many terminally ill patients and should not be withheld if it will so relieve incontinence and other symptoms that the patient can remain at home.

BLOOD TRANSFUSION

Chronic anaemia is common in advanced disease, particularly malignancy. Many of its features mimic those of the malignancy itself, such as dyspnoea, drowsiness, confusion, angina, pallor, lethargy, palpitations. It is often not easy to know how much suffering is due to the anaemia and therefore whether or not a transfusion might help. The following guidelines are suggested.

1. Ask the patient whether past transfusions have helped and in what way. A remarkably high proportion will describe feeling better after earlier transfusions but not more recent ones, though most will say the doctors felt the transfusion had been useful! If a patient whose opinion can be relied upon says he or she felt no different after a transfusion, it is not worth giving another one.
2. The only symptoms ever likely to be eased by a transfusion of red cell concentrate are dyspnoea (if the anaemia appears to be the principal cause of it), and angina but the latter is understandably uncommon in the patients we are discussing in this context.

3. A haemoglobin level above 8 g does not need a transfusion.
4. The patient and relatives must be left in no doubt why a transfusion is, or is not, being given. Knowing that transfusions may be life-saving after haemorrhages at other times in life, many patients need help to understand why they are anaemic, that not having a blood transfusion is not condemning them to die and, conversely, giving them blood is not aimed at maintaining life in the presence of a life-threatening condition such as malignancy.

Obvious as it may be, it merits repeating—a blood transfusion should not be given to 'make the patient feel better' or to help the doctor feel he is 'doing something'. The strong impression from palliative care units where transfusions of red cell concentrate are often given is that many fewer patients than expected seem to benefit from them.

BREATHLESSNESS

Like pain, breathlessness is anticipated and feared, especially by the patient found to have a primary or secondary lung malignancy. The possibility of a slow death from asphyxia crosses the mind of many patients. However, whereas in pain there is much we can do, there is disappointingly little for some of the conditions and complications which lead to progressive breathlessness. This is especially so when two or more conditions are superimposed as with bronchogenic carcinoma on longstanding chronic obstructive pulmonary disease or lymphangitis carcinomatosis in the patient with chronic cardiac insufficiency.

Some of the principal causes of breathlessness are illustrated in Figure 2.1. They will be dealt with in this section in alphabetical order, but it must be remembered that each will be only one piece of a kaleidoscope of symptoms, the overall clinical picture being that of steadily increasing incapacity and mental anguish if it is not skilfully dealt with.

Non-specific treatment

1. Attempt to modify the pathological processes where possible.
2. Opioids are the best drugs we have to reduce tachypnoea and anxiety. Correctly used on a regular basis, they do not suppress respiration and can be shown to improve it. The secret is to use the smallest effective dose, *regularly*, remembering that with the opioids renal function is more important than hepatic function, and the younger the patient the higher the dose required. A good rule is to start with aqueous morphine 2.5 milligram every 4 hours, increasing if necessary to 5 milligram every 4 hours. If the patient is already on an opioid agonist for analgesia, 30–50 per cent more should be prescribed to control dyspnoea. When the dose requirement has been defined, the prescription can be changed to MST for convenience.

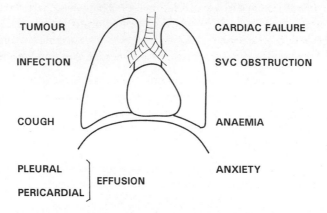

NEURO-MUSCULAR

TUMOUR

INFECTION

COUGH

PLEURAL
        } EFFUSION
PERICARDIAL

CARDIAC FAILURE

SVC OBSTRUCTION

ANAEMIA

ANXIETY

ELEVATION OF DIAPHRAGM

Fig. 2.1 Common causes of breathlessness.

3. Anxiolytics are occasionally needed even with opioids. For immediate short-term relief, use lorazepam 0.5−1 milligram sublingually. For more protracted effect, use diazepam 2−10 milligram each night.

4. Panic attacks are almost inevitable and must be treated energetically and effectively if the patient is not to lose faith in his carers. Try either:

   • lorazepam 0.5−1 milligram sublingually or
   • midazolam 2.5−5 milligram subcutaneously as detailed on p. 26 or
   • Diazemuls 5−10 milligram intravenously as detailed elsewhere.

5. Oxygen is only indicated, as at any other time, for anoxia and not as a placebo, as a means of keeping a dying patient alive, or to resuscitate someone almost dead—all popular misunderstandings of the lay public. It is important for the family doctor to appreciate that inappropriate prescribing of domiciliary oxygen makes a family feel that the patient's life depends on it and if, for any reason, it is not beside the patient day and night (as might be so in hospital) they soon request hospital admission when that patient might easily have been cared for at home.

CONFUSION

At some time or other in their terminal illness, close to 40 per cent of patients will suffer confusion. In hospitals and palliative care units their care can be difficult, but at home their confusional state can soon constitute a crisis threatening the resolve to nurse them at home. Relatives are often willing to look after a loved one in pain or experiencing dyspnoea, incontinence, and many other symptoms, but few are prepared for confusion. It is important, therefore, to anticipate this problem and forewarn the carers that it may occur and promise that both doctor and nurse will work closely together and with the family to help correct or contain it. If carers are not warned that it might develop, they soon assume it is medication-induced — something the doctor should not have allowed to happen — and confidence can soon be lost.

Causes (see Table 2.3)

Management

1. Review all possible causes and treat appropriately. If confusion has developed as an *acute* event, the most likely causes are:

   - infection (upper respiratory tract infection (URTI), urinary tract infection (UTI), chest, bedsore)
   - distended bladder
   - impacted rectum
   - hypoxia
   - metabolic (especially hypercalcaemia, hyponatraemia, or acute-on-chronic renal failure).

2. Review all medication, reducing or discontinuing if possible, any likely causative agents, checking up on any past history of drug reactions or unusual adverse effects. In particular, look at:

   - steroids
   - H_2 antagonists
   - benzodiazepines.

3. Review the opioids in use. Though most patients can take adequate doses of opioid without being confused, the occasional patient is encountered where confusion clears immediately on changing to a different type and dose of opioid. Morphine or diamorphine might, for example, be changed to methadone, fentanyl, or phenazocine.

   Sometimes the problem is caused by bolus injections and corrected by giving the same 24-hour dose more slowly and steadily by subcutaneous infusion via a syringe-driver. It is, however, vitally important for a doctor and nurse to be agreed on such changes and be able to speak with one voice to relatives who otherwise may assume the original prescription was wrong or even dangerous, or that pain will now recur as a result of opioid change.

4. Consider a neuroleptic. For younger patients the preferable one is haloperidol, 1.5–5 milligram per day in single daily doses unless rapid sedation is needed when SC or even IV haloperidol can be given in 5 milligram doses.

Table 2.3 *Potentially correctable causes of confusion*

Raised intracranial pressure
  primary brain tumour
  secondary brain tumour

Hypoxia

Infection (in any system, with or without pyrexia)

Drug-induced
  Anticholinergic drugs
  Benzodiazepines
  CNS stimulants
  H_2 antagonists
  Opioids
  Phenothiazines
  Steroids

Metabolic
  Hypercalcaemia
  Hyponatraemia
  Uraemia (prerenal, renal or postrenal)
  Hepatic failure (acute or chronic)
  Hypo- or hyperglycaemia
  Hypothyroidism

Psychotic reaction to illness

Anaemia
  Iron deficiency
  B_{12} deficiency

Constipation

Urinary retention

Depressive state

Withdrawal of alcohol or drug after longterm dependency

The young patient with disruptive, aggressive behaviour (for example, with a glioma or brain damage) will need pericyazine as described on pp. 27 and 49. For elderly patients, thioridazine is preferable, 10–25 milligram three times a day. Both haloperidol and thioridazine are preferable to the phenothiazines because they have fewer anticholinergic effects, but excellent sedation can be achieved in the bedbound patient with methotrimeprazine 25–50 milligram three times a day. Its hypotensive effect makes it a hazardous drug for the ambulant patient.

Many doctors prefer to use benzodiazepines for their sedative effects but care must be exercised. In many people, confusion can be exacerbated with benzodiazepines and drugs such as SC midazolam; whilst undoubtedly valuable for immediate short-term sedation, they are also amnesiogenic, making the patient even more confused, disorientated, and distressed when the drug wears off. Having said that, there is probably no better drug than midazolam in a syringe-driver (combined if necessary with the opioid) for the patient near to death.

5. Non-drug measures should be considered. The patient should be cared for in a familiar, safe environment, not moved from room to room or separated from familiar objects. Carers and visitors should be restricted where possible to the most familiar and 'unthreatening' behaviour. A good deal can be achieved with a background of much loved music, the same level of lighting on all the time, intrusive background noises excluded.

It is absolutely *essential*, that all members of the family are informed about confusion and its possible causes, leaving them in no doubt that it is a result of the illness and not a major psychiatric development. The family should be shown how to speak to the patient and to respond to his questions, how to maintain a peaceful and unthreatening atmosphere, and how to exclude unwanted, unhelpful visitors whose presence may make matters worse.

Admission to hospital or palliative care unit may become necessary but should be a last resort because it will entail a move to new surroundings and new attendants. When a patient is near to death, it often becomes necessary to accede to the pleas of relatives that the patient be heavily sedated if he is to stay at home under their care.

CONSTIPATION

Next to aesthenia, this is the most common problem requiring palliation in the terminally ill. It is more common than pain, yet gets less attention and when it does its management is seldom rational and well planned. Doctors leave it to nurses and nurses often deal with it without any rational or validated protocol. Soon everyone is frustrated, not least the patient who takes the symptom more seriously than anyone else.

Causes

The causes are well known to all the professionals and most patients but rarely amenable to change. Diet cannot be changed much and the introduction of high fibre food will rarely be acceptable to these patients, important as it is earlier in life. Many of the drugs they must take, particularly the opioids, are constipating and these patients become less active and drink less fluid.

Short of prescribing appropriate laxatives, what can be done? If a non-constipating drug can usefully be substituted for a constipating one, this should be done but it has to be remembered that most of the strong opioids have little to choose between them in this respect. Most patients can be encouraged to take a higher fluid intake and some will agree to orange or tomato juice first thing in the morning. Toasted wholemeal bread can be encouraged.

It cannot be overemphasized that prior to prescribing any laxative, whether oral or rectal, a rectal examination must be performed. If this rule was always followed, there would be fewer patients suffering spurious diarrhoea, enduring nausea because of gross colonic loading, and going in and out of subacute intestinal obstruction.

Rectal examination and assessment

Filled with hard faeces Do not give either a faecal expander (which will only convert a small hard mass into a large soft one, impossible to expel and equally difficult to remove manually) or a peristaltic stimulant until the hard faeces have been broken up. Prescribe a warm, Arachis oil (or olive oil) enema at night for two successive nights, and either two bisacodyl suppositories or a phosphate enema in the mornings. Only when further rectal examination shows that the rectal mass has been expelled, and the contents are now soft, can the main-tenance laxative be selected and prescribed.

Empty ballooned rectum This indicates faecal impaction high in the rectum or at the sigmorectal junction. Do not give a faecal expander (which will only worsen the high impaction) unless it is accompanied by a peristaltic stimulant to encourage the softened mass to descend into the rectum. Do not give either enemata or suppositories, unlikely to help but certain to irritate the empty rectum and further worry or embarrass the patient. Prescribe a peristaltic stimulant (senna, bisacodyl), and either a high-dose osmotic laxative (lactulose) or a faecal expander (Docusate). Daily rectal examination is mandatory to ensure that the mass which has moved down from higher up is not now producing rectal impaction where it will need the Arachis oil regimen described.

Empty collapsed rectum There is no impaction in either rectum or sigmorectal junction. Careful abdominal examination is called for to identify loaded sigmoid or descending colon. There is no need for energetic rectal treatment unless oral laxatives cannot be given. Thought must be given to an appropriate 'main-tenance' regimen.

Laxative routine

The choice of laxative once the rectum has been emptied will depend on:

• the patient's ability to take tablets or liquids
• the underlying pathology, whether the bowel is at risk, or there could develop subacute obstruction

- the fluid intake (if poor, osmotic laxatives will be ineffective)
- other drugs being taken (and particularly the opioids).

It is worth remembering the laxative group and their salient features.

1. *Lubricant laxatives:* Liquid paraffin is the only one, effective after a latency period of 1—3 days, but likely to produce lipoid pneumonia if aspirated. It is not recommended even as the emulsion.
2. *Faecal softener laxatives:* These include docusate sodium and poloximer— neither of which often used alone. More popular and useful are codanthrusate and codanthramer.
3. *Osmotic laxatives:* These include lactulose, sorbitol and mannitol. It is difficult to know why lactulose is so much prescribed. Terminally ill patients seldom like its sickly taste, rarely have sufficient fluid intake to make it work, and in the doses often required (but seldom prescribed) there can be bloating and colic. It is very expensive and better preparations are available. Magnesium salts are also osmotic but peristaltic stimulants. Sulphate salt is too drastic for most patients but magnesium hydroxide can be recommended.
4. *Peristaltic stimulant laxatives*: These include senna, danthron, bisacodyl and sodium picosulphate. All are capable of producing colic and faecal incontinence in the very frail but can usefully and logically be combined with an osmotic laxative such as lactulose or magnesium hydroxide.

Whatever is prescribed, try to change the regimen as seldom as possible in the hope that the patient will not alternate between near impaction (with or without spurious diarrhoea) and diarrhoeal incontinence.

No matter how rewarding the result of rectal treatment, nurses in particular should avoid the temptation to keep giving suppositories and/or enemata. It is better to discuss the problem with the doctor, decide on a rational oral regimen, and plan who is to be responsible for the regular reviews. Factors which may necessitate changes in the routine include:

- an increase in opioid dose (usually necessitating an increase in laxatives)
- the introduction to prokinetic drugs (metoclopramide, domperidone and cisapride) which may improve peristalsis
- changes in fluid intake and loss.

The management of constipation demands as much skilled cooperation between doctor and community nurses as the management of pain.

COUGH

Although bronchogenic carcinoma and lung secondaries from many other malignancies and chronic bronchitis are common, cough is not a common

problem. There is much which can be done to help and what is described here
is as appropriate for chronic obstructive pulmonary disease as for malignancy.

Causes

- bronchial obstruction due to primary or secondary tumour, or mediastinal
  adenopathy
- lymphangitis carcinomatosis
- secondary bronchial infection, penumonia or infection in a necrotic tumour
- left ventricular failure (LVF) with characteristic cough and dyspnoea wakening the patient.

Management of a productive cough

1. The role of the physiotherapist in aiding expectoration and drainage is pre-
   eminent. This may be a utopian dream in most homes but when one is
   available a physiotherapist should be called in, even if only to teach the
   patient, family carers, and community nurses what to do.
2. Antibiotics (as described elsewhere) are helpful in clearing infection and so
   reducing sputum. If no sensitivities can be done, it is justifiable to give a
   short course of a broad spectrum antibiotic to relieve the cough.
3. Mucolytics (e.g. bromhexine 8–16 milligram three times a day) are occasionally useful but only when used regularly for a minimum of four weeks.

Management of a dry, unproductive cough

1. Cough suppressants such as codeine or pholcodeine linctus (10 ml 4-hourly),
   methadone linctus (2 milligram 4- or 6-hourly), or immediate action morphine (2.5 milligram 4-hourly) can be useful. If the patient is already on a
   strong opioid for analgesia, the dose to suppress non-productive cough
   should be increased by 50 per cent and then returned to the analgesic dose
   as soon as the cough is relieved.
2. Humidification of the atmosphere is particularly useful in centrally- or gas-
   heated rooms. At home the doctor will suggest a bowl of water in front of
   the fire if there is one or suggest a steam kettle in the bedroom until the
   dryness has been dispelled. The best method is to provide a nebulizer, instruct in its use, and nebulize 'water for injection' or saline every 4 hours.
3. Steroids (dexamethasone 2–4 milligram each morning) will reduce oedema
   surrounding a tumour or in the bronchi but are not likely to have much
   success in relieving bronchospasm at this stage.
4. Bupivacaine (2 ml of 0.25 per cent solution) nenbulized every 4 or 6 hours
   is probably the most consistently successful method known. It is essential for
   the patient to breath normally and not try to take deep breaths, and to take

no food or fluid for thirty minutes at least after each treatment because of the suppression of cough reflexes by the anaesthetic.

Correct positioning of the patient is important. Contrary to what people think, patients with bronchogenic carcinoma prefer not to be nursed bold-upright and during sleep are often to be found comfortable with neither cough nor dyspnoea on only two or three pillows. The patient with chronic obstructive pulmonary disease must be nursed as upright as possible and the one with the pleural effusion should lie on the affected side so as not to produce mediastinal shift.

DEATH RATTLE

This is one of those uncommon instances where the patient, almost always unconscious, is treated for the sake of the relatives. No matter how unaware of the noise the patient clearly is, relatives are usually distressed, fearing the patient is drowning in his own secretions, or 'fighting for breath'. Time spent in explaining it to the relatives is never wasted. Even better is for the doctor or nurse to anticipate it, explaining in advance when the patient is becoming more frail and drowsy both what Cheyne-Stokes respiration will be like (and its significance) and the 'death rattle' itself.

Management

Anticipation is the axiom here. When secretions have already collected in the throat, only time or suction will clear them. It is better to give something to prevent it happening, but the timing can be difficult.

1. Hyoscine hydrobromide, 0.4–0.6 milligram every 4 hours, can be given subcutaneously. Rather than so many injections, it is preferable to use a syringe-driver (particularly if it is already in use or being considered for diamorphine infusion) in which case the 24-hour requirement of 2.4 or 3.6 milligram is used, compatible with either morphine or diamorphine in the syringe-driver, provided the mixture is reconstituted daily.
2. Hyoscine transdermal patches (Scopoderm) are expensive but more comfortable and acceptable for many patients, being placed behind the ear and changed every 72 hours.

   Naturally, all exogenous secretions will be reduced, making oral hygiene even more important, any sputum more viscid, and constipation worse but by this stage the latter may not matter. Much more serious can be the confusion sometimes produced with hyoscine, sometimes bordering on the psychotic. In this case, the drug must be discontinued and replaced with glycopyrrolate 0.2 milligram every 8 or 12 hours. For some reason this drug is sometimes effective when hyoscine was not. The frequency of administration is dictated by response. There are no data on its use in a syringe-driver.

3. There is no place for tricyclic antidepressants or any other anticholinergic drug other than those mentioned for this problem.

DEPRESSION

This is a common problem but difficult to treat. There are several reasons for this.

We are all keen not to medicalize an appropriate reaction to an illness and no one can doubt that having a fatal illness affecting every aspect of life must be depressing. It must be more so if suffering which can be palliated is not handled appropriately, or if anxieties and misunderstandings build up because of insensitive or conflicting advice and comments from the professionals. It is clearly important to differentiate depression from sadness but when does one merge into the other sufficient to merit treatment?

The cardinal symptoms of a depressive state are well known but most are also the features of terminal illness, particularly if it is a protracted one—poor sleep pattern, poor concentration, a sense of hopelessness, feeling a burden on others, loss of appetite and energy, a sense of guilt, and so on. Should every such patient be put onto antidepressants?

We all know the unpleasant adverse effects of the tricyclics and the long time which elapses before benefit is seen. Side-effects are certainly less with the newer families of antidepressants but there is still a delay before the suffering patient feels it has been worth taking yet another tablet. Is the answer to start them early or to hold off as long as possible in the hope that good symptom palliation will obviate the need for antidepressants, running the risk that if they are eventually needed much time will have been wasted? Current thinking is as follows:

1. Sadness is different from a depressive state and should not be treated with antidepressants.
2. Much depression is related to poorly controlled suffering, particularly physical and psychological, and no effort should be spared in addressing this problem.
3. The presence of a disturbed or altered sleep pattern (unless caused by poorly controlled pain) should lead to the suspicion of depression and appropriate treatment. This is especially so in cases where the disturbed sleep is accompanied by features of apathy, poor concentration, or a sense of being a burden on others.
4. The first line antidepressants which should be tried are fluoxetine taken in the morning, or trazadone at night because of its marked sedative properties. It must be remembered, however, that fluoxetine can produce

nausea, transient anxiety, and appetite suppression which may last for several weeks, and that with its active metabolites its half-life is 7−14 days.

5. The second line drugs should be the older tricyclics in lower doses than would be used in the physically healthy (for example, 25−125 milligram amitriptyline daily). Amitriptyline or doxepin is best for the agitated depressed patient with insomnia, and desipramine or nortriptyline (being relatively non-anticholinergic) preferable where one must avoid exacerbating urinary retention, decreased intestinal motility, or stomatitis.

6. There is no place for the monoamine oxidase inhibitors (MAOIs) or stimulants such as amphetamine except in the hands of psychiatrists experienced with this group of patients.

Members of the primary care team and lay carers may be anxious in case the patient attempts suicide, particularly when he has expressed suicidal thoughts. What meagre research has been done on suicide in terminally ill patients suggests that suicide attempts are very rare, almost always associated with premorbid psychopathology and/or often a long recognized personality disorder, manifesting itself in hysterical, manipulative behaviour. It is therefore possible to say with some confidence, and possibly to many people's surprise, that for the vast majority of these terminally ill patients suicide attempts or suicidal ideas are rare. When they do occur—in those with pre-existing psychopathology or personality disorder—they are cries for help rather than attempts to end life.

DIARRHOEA

True diarrhoea is uncommon in the terminally ill, affecting only 4 per cent of patients in palliative care units. Many are admitted because of it but it later turns out to be spurious, the result of neglected (and often iatrogenic) faecal impaction. On the other hand, diarrhoea is a major problem in AIDS.

Causes

1. *Spurious—due to faecal impaction*: Every patient needs a careful rectal examination no matter how graphically he describes the diarrhoea. If in any doubt it is always worth having a straight X-ray of abdomen done. When the radiologist knows what is being considered and finds loading, he may offer to do a gastrographin enema which will both help to define colonic pathology and act as an excellent laxative. It is a safe rule in palliative care that all diarrhoea is spurious, due to constipation, until proved otherwise and no antidiarrhoea preparations should be prescribed until impaction and colonic loading have been excluded.

2. *Infection, as at any other time of life*: Cryptosporidiosis may be the cause in about one-third of AIDS patients with diarrhoea. In these patients salmonella

may not be controllable but diarrhoea due to cytomegalovirus colitis can be treated.

3. *Inflammatory bowel disease (Crohn's, colitis, diverticulitis* etc.,): this should also be considered.
4. *Internal fistulae (e.g. ileocolic, colocolic)*: This is suspected when diarrhoea develops acutely, no organisms are found, no loading is seen on straight films, and no antidiarrhoea agents help. Such fistulae are tragic complications of colonic and bladder carcinoma but seldom seen in ovarian malignancy.
5. *Excessive laxatives (medically or self-prescribed) or, less commonly, the result of prokinetic drugs such as metoclopramide, domperidone, or cisapride*: Many self-medicating patients, disillusioned with our laxatives, their volume and unattractive flavour, resort to over-the-counter preparations containing phenolthalene in a chocolate base.

Management

Uncontrollable diarrhoea in a person thought to have many weeks or even months to live, merits admission to hospital or palliative care unit. It should never become the terminal event in a patient's life. This is particularly the case with AIDS. Treat anything treatable—over-enthusiastic laxatives, infection, antibiotic-induced diarrhoea, cytomegalovirus colitis.

1. Loperamide can be prescribed 4 milligram as required. Uniquely, this drug can be taken intermittently after each diarrhoeal bowel action, has a speedy action, and can regularize the bowel function rather than simply constipating. Most respond to 4 milligram four times a day but occasionally one must give it every 4 hours.
2. Diphenoxylate 5 milligram three times a day is probably less useful than loperamide and can produce dry mouth, drowsiness, and lightheadedness. In elderly patients it can produce confusional state and should be avoided.
3. Codeine phosphate 30–60 milligram three times a day should be used cautiously. It produces loculation of the faeces and the patient quickly moves from liquid faeces to hard 'golf-balls' very likely to produce rectal impaction and spurious diarrhoea.
4. Pancreatic extracts taken with meals readily control steatorrhoea, itself often mistaken for diarrhoea by patients and feared because the greasy stools adhering to toilet pans are thought by them to be infectious or carriers of pancreatic cancer. It must be remembered that these pancreatic extracts can worsen nausea and anorexia. Cholestyramine used to relieve pruritus due to obstructive jaundice worsens steatorrhoea.
5. Methylcellulose, in tablet or granule form, remains one of the most useful agents for bowel regularizing in patients with diverticular disease, often

increasingly troublesome when they can no longer manage the traditional high roughage diet.

6. Octreotide, a somatostatin analogue, is capable of controlling even the most intractable diarrhoea. It needs to be started in the hospital or palliative care unit by injection and at considerable cost.

DYSPHAGIA

Different studies report the incidence of dysphagia in the terminally ill as being between 12 and 23 per cent. What matters is that it is a more common symptom than might have been thought.

Causes

1. Pharyngeal obstruction resulting from intrinsic pressure from tumour, oedema, infection or extrinsic pressure from tumour and nodes;
2. Oesophageal candidiasis, producing a picture of painful rather than difficult swallowing, with symptoms resembling hiatus hernia or acid reflux;
3. Oesophageal obstruction, intrinsically from carcinoma, stenosis, or blocked Celestin or Atkinson tube, or extrinsically from enlarged mediastinal nodes or, much less commonly, pleural effusion;
4. Neuromuscular dysfunction, as in motor neurone disease and some of the rarer myopathies.

Management

1. Treat the primary cause where possible. This may be antifungals for candidiasis, radiotherapy or chemotherapy for nodes exerting extrinsic pressure etc. Radiation mucositis will settle spontaneously but relief can be obtained with antacid/surface anaesthetic preparations, indomethacin (proven effective in such cases), benzydamine gargle (15 millilitres) every 4 hours, or carbenoxolone.
2. Celestin or Atkinson tubes can be invaluable for a carcinoma of the lower third of the oesophagus. The patient should be shown one to appreciate the size of its lumen, be instructed to take a liquidized diet, and 'anything you would normally eat with a spoon', be forbidden to each white bread, hard or dry food, and sandwiches of any description. Before each meal he should take a teaspoon of honey in a little warm water and a mouthful of an aerated drink of any sort before, after, and frequently during each meal, irrespective of its content. The sudden recurrence of dysphagia in such a patient almost always signifies a blockage of the tube with a food bolus. Very occasionally it will clear with copious fizzy drinks. More usually it needs endoscopic

clearing and a firm reminder to the patient of the dietary restrictions and rules.

3. Laser therapy is becoming increasingly available and can reduce the bulk of an oesophageal carcinoma or maintain a modest lumen after the first day or so when the dysphagia is temporarily worse.

4. Dexamethasone (8 milligram each morning reducing as quickly as possible to 2 milligram daily) can be effective in relieving mediastinal adenopathy not amenable to radiotherapy or chemotherapy.

5. Skilled nursing care can ensure good oral hygiene and hydration, the patient being given a plentiful supply of ice and iced fluids, taught the correct positioning after meals, and advised to use flexi straws to reduce air swallowing.

FAECAL INCONTINENCE

Though urinary incontinence will often be tolerated at home, faecal incontinence usually leads to a request for admission, even when the primary care team has sufficient nursing time to offer and the back-up of a special laundry service. Energetic investigation and treatment are essential.

Causes

1. Lax anal sphincter, particularly in the elderly and very frail from any cause
2. Faecal impaction and spurious diarrhoea
3. Excessive laxatives, particularly the peristaltic stimulants, and preparations containing liquid paraffin
4. Anorectal carcinoma, particularly if there is a mucous discharge.

Management

1. Every effort should be made to find the cause. The patient with a lax sphincter will not benefit from pelvic floor exercises but from an agent to firm up the stool, for example loperamide, methylcellulose, or codeine phosphate. The constipated patient needs attention as outlined in this book on p.36.

2. The unfortunate patient with an anorectal carcinoma may be helped by:

   (a) radiotherapy, particularly if it is fungating or bleeding
   (b) laser therapy
   (c) rectal steroids (prednisolone suppositories twice a day or retention enemata daily or betamethasone foam twice a day)
   (d) incontinence pads (it is remarkable how many patients improvise something when pads could be prescribed)
   (e) an air freshener.

3. By the time the patient has faecal incontinence, the condition may be too advanced to benefit from it, but it is always worth seeking a surgical opinion on fashioning a defunctioning colostomy unless there is a heavy mucous leak from a carcinoma.
4. Paraplegic patients, and some with motor neurone disease, are helped by being made constipated and having twice- or thrice-weekly manual evacuations. Clearly, the last thing they want is a peristaltic stimulant which will only produce colic and incontinence, or a faecal softener which will make manual evacuation impossible.

FUNGATING TUMOURS AND ODOURS

Here we are looking particularly at the problems of bleeding and malodours, not the puzzling array of topical dressings which are available but are so often used empirically rather than scientifically.

Capillary bleeding from a fungating tumour or pressure sore can be reduced by applying:

- haemostatic dressings such as Kaltostat
- silver nitrate soaks applied daily in a strength of 1:5000, made up specially and kept in a dark bottle
- adrenalin soaks in the strength of 1:1000
- Oxycel or Polycel gauze (difficult to obtain but the most effective)
- Alum paste 1 per cent to the site
- bismuth subnitrate/iodoform paste (BIPP) applied generously on gauze pressed firmly on the tumour and changed every 3 or 4 days.

Malodour can be reduced with:

- metronidazole gel applied daily direct to the site (if unobtainable, metronidazole pessaries can be shaved, ground down and mixed with KY Jelly to make the application)
- bismuth subnitrate/iodoform paste (BIPP) re-applied every 3 or 4 days
- activated charcoal pads (Denidor, Actasorb) applied over all the other dressings and changed daily.

Exudates can be reduced with:

- absorbent dressings such as Kaltostat or Debrisan
- honey or icing sugar applied directly to the site.

It should not be forgotten that radiotherapy can sometimes help fungating lesions and that surgical debridement to remove all necrotic tumour aids the application and effectiveness of medications as well as reducing odour.

HALITOSIS

Rarely do terminally ill people mention this but, being a source of embarrassment to them and to relatives, it should be treated where possible.

Causes

1. Diseases of the mouth and poor oral hygiene—gingivitis, stomatitis, dental sepsis, ulceration and candidiasis;
2. Diseases of the respiratory tract—infections of sinuses, tonsils, lungs (especially chronic bronchiectasis and lung abscess) and necrotic bronchogenic carcinomata;
3. Diseases of the digestive tract—hiatus hernia, gastric stasis or stagnation ('cesspool halitosis') often due to carcinoma and particularly linitus plastica;
4. Metabolic failure—diabetic ketoacidosis, uraemia, hepatic insufficiency.

Whilst in healthy people, one must also look to incriminate foods such as garlic, onions, radishes, curry etc., this is unlikely to be the cause in the terminally ill.

Management

Where possible, specific treatment should be given if a cause can be identified. Otherwise, peppermint or Double Amplex in conjunction with the following:

- scrupulous attention to oral hygiene (something relatives can do)
- prokinetic drugs (metoclopramide and cisapride) for gastric stasis
- broad spectrum antibiotics for chest infections whilst awaiting sputum bacteriology reports and sensitivity
- oral metronidazole 200 milligram three times a day, even when no sensitive organism can be identified.

HICCUP

Distressing, persistent hiccup is much more common in women than in men. Studies have shown it is usually of psychogenic origin in women but, in both sexes, the following checklist should be followed.

Causes

1. Irritation of the phrenic nerve anywhere in its course but particularly by tumour at the hilum of the lung;
2. Irritation of the diaphragm by tumour or infection;

3. Uraemia;
4. Dyspepsia, especially with hiatus hernia, gastric stasis and aerophagy (with uraemia, the commonest cause in the terminally ill);
5. Elevation of the diaphragm as a result of hepatomegaly, ascites, or subphrenic masses;
6. Raised intracranial pressure or cerebrovascular disease, the latter being the most common cause in the non-terminally ill, especially the aged.

Management

1. Correct the underlying cause. This is seldom possible except for uraemia, chest infection, and after successful radiation of mediastinal adenopathy.
2. Re-breathing CO_2 from a paper or plastic bag is the traditional remedy and effective in minor cases, but sometimes an alarming procedure for the very frail.
3. Pharyngeal stimulation involves inserting a nasal catheter 8−12 cm into the nose so that it is opposite the second cervical vertebrae when it is then gently pushed in and out, usually with immediate cessation of hiccup. Of course, it frequently recurs after this treatment.
4. All of the following drugs have been tried and can be recommended:

   (a) a defoaming antiflatulent before and after each meal, preferable to the traditional peppermint water for those with gastric distension;
   (b) chlorpromazine 10−25 milligram orally three times a day, giving as low a dose as possible in the elderly (very rarely is an intravenous injection needed);
   (c) prokinetic drugs (metoclopramide, domperidone and cisapride) for gastric distension;
   (d) baclofen 5 milligram twice daily, but doses as high as 20 milligram three times daily have been used;
   (e) amantadine;
   (f) nefidipine 10−20 milligram three times a day;
   (g) glucogen, if the hiccup is caused by distension of the gall bladder secondary to opioid-induced constriction of the Sphincter of Oddi;
   (h) phrenic crush, once a recommended option, is never necessary in these patients.

HYPERCALCAEMIA

Estimates vary but this complication of cancer occurs in 5−10 per cent of patients, predominantly but not exclusively in those with squamous cell tumour whether of bronchus, cervix, oesophagus, or any other site. Though often associated with bone metastases, hypercalcaemia can occur when few if any bone secondaries are known. The condition is often overlooked as is the treatment which can restore a good quality of life.

Hypercalcaemia should be suspected in any patient with:

- a squamous cell carcinoma
- a sudden onset of confusion or vagueness
- polydipsia and polyuria
- rapidly worsening lethargy, listlessness, apathy, and generalized flaccidity.

Clearly these same features could be those of any advanced malignancy, making it essential for the doctor to have a high level of suspicion and a readiness to take blood for plasma calcium and albumin estimation (always remembering to remove the tourniquet before taking the specimen).

Management

In those with a corrected calcium level of 2.5–3.0 mmol/l, it may be sufficient to increase oral fluid intake and keep the situation under review. If there are no contraindications to their use, steroids can be given: dexamethasone 4–6 milligram each morning until normocalcaemia is achieved.

If the corrected calcium is over 3.0 mmol/l, it is preferable for the patient to be admitted to hospital or palliative care unit for IV saline rehydration and an IV bisphosphonate such as pamidronate. There is usually both subjective and biochemical improvement within 72 hours and normocalcaemia may be maintained without further IV bisphosphonates for 21–28 days, but it is now more usual practice to maintain most patients on oral bisphosphonates, regularly checking the biochemistry once normocalcaemia has been achieved with IV pamidronate.

When possible, specific treatment is given to the underlying malignancy, either by radiotherapy or, when appropriate, chemotherapy, with the intention of reducing the secretion of the parathormone-like substance causing the hypercalcaemia.

Contrary to what some people used to believe, the withholding of milk is not necessary in these patients. Left untreated, severe hypercalcaemia (i.e. over 3.5 mmol/l) can lead to death within a week or so.

INSOMNIA

At least 70 per cent of terminally ill patients will report insomnia. It not only troubles them but also affects relatives looking after them who feel sleep is essential and are very conscious of not getting sufficient sleep themselves. It does not take many wakeful nights before exhausted carers begin to ask if hospitalization might not be better for the patient.

Causes

1. Physical distresses such as pain, pruritus, cough and dyspnoea, bedsores, or urinary frequency;
2. Depression, so characteristically altering the sleep pattern, most frequently showing as early morning wakening but in others as shallow sleep with frequent wakening and feeling exhausted by the morning;
3. Hallucinations and nightmares, occasionally evidence of psychotic derangement but often caused by such benzodiazepines as nitrazepam or the H_2-antagonists cimetidine and ranitidine, and steroids taken late in the day;
4. Cerebral pathology, such as glioma, when the patient seems to turn night into day and vice-versa;
5. Anxiety, where the patient cannot get off to sleep because of worries and fears which continue to bother them whenever they waken;
6. Nightsweats, particularly in patients with hepatic metastases and the occasional patient with chronic infection such as tuberculosis and the opportunistic infections of AIDS;
7. Drug withdrawal in a patient long dependent on benzodiazepines, opioids, or alcohol which have recently been reduced or discontinued.

Management

1. Search for, and treat appropriately, all physical causes. Most have been described in this book but prime attention should be paid to pain so often described as worse at night. It is important to realize that pain at night is nearly always organic and, conversely, pain described as severe during the day but not sufficient to waken the patient or prevent them getting off to sleep is almost always psychogenic—in need of skilled attention but not necessarily an analgesic.
2. Explore all anxieties and carefully exclude depression. The patient who has no other features of depression yet cannot sleep may still have a treatable depressive state but is more likely to have unventilated or unaddressed fears. Paradoxically, doctors and nurses can be the cause of such insomnia. With the best of intentions, we so often explain to terminally ill patients how peaceful death can be—'just like a good sleep'—that they dread falling asleep in case they die that night. They seem to will themselves to stay awake.
3. Exclude disturbances caused by drugs. If nitrazepam is implicated, change to another sedative such as thioridazine or pericyazine. If due to diuresis, change the time when diuretics are taken. Reference is often made in this book to the correct timing of dexamethasone administration. Very frequently this is forgotten and the patient allowed to take the dexamethasone late in the afternoon or evening with the predictable result that they are stimulated and suffer not only wakefulness but agitation and fear.

4. Treat nightsweats as described in this text.
5. Reverse the disturbed sleep pattern of the glioma patient by giving high-dose pericyazine at night to ensure a good sleep, then cut back the dose when benefit shows. In younger patients, doses as high as 30 milligram will be needed initially, with proportionately smaller doses in older, frailer patients.
6. Give adequate doses of any sedative rather than modest doses which may only produce confused, light sleep and further anxiety about this insomnia. It is worth remembering that when high doses of opioids are needed for pain, proportionately higher doses of benzodiazepines, phenothiazines, and butyl-phenones will also be needed for these patients. The patient who previously took diazepam 2 milligram may now need 10–20 milligram, the patient on temazepam 10 milligram now needing 20–30 milligram, and so on.
7. Check that all environmental factors have been corrected. Some will need a night-light left on, or a background of favourite music specially recorded on a longplaying tape for them. Those with respiratory conditions such as chronic obstructive pulmonary disease, cardiac failure, or bronchogenic carcinoma may find it better to spend the night in an armchair (usually against the advice and instinct of their relatives) and all should be reminded that late-night TV thrillers are not conducive to sleep.

In short, insomnia is a major problem worthy of considerable attention to every detail rather than the automatic prescription of a doctor's favourite hypnotic. A person who is able to get a good sleep is likely to have more comfortable days and be able to stay at home longer. Conversely, the one whose strength and resolve are diminished by insomnia soon ends up in hospital or hospice.

INTESTINAL OBSTRUCTION

Though the diagnosis of this relatively common condition in the terminally ill cancer patient is not difficult, its management certainly is. It is particularly difficult for the family doctor who has to decide whether he should and can manage it conservatively at home or have the patient admitted with all that that entails.

Gastric outlet obstruction

If the obstruction is a high one, near the gastric outlet, the patient will keep nothing down, have minimal nausea and often report feeling better after each sudden unexpected vomit. There will be minimal pain and no colic. That patient, irrespective of the primary diagnosis, requires admission to hospital for naso-gastric suction to decompress the stomach, IV fluids, and electrolytes, and attempts to relieve the cause of the gastric outlet obstruction. The key questions to be asked by the family doctor are, 'Do you feel sick all the time?' and 'Do you actually feel better when you have vomited?'.

Intestinal obstruction

The person who is known to have abdominal pathology capable of producing acute or subacute obstruction (and therefore does not need investigations and/or laparotomy to diagnose it) does not need 'drip and suction' as a routine. In fact, he can be cared for at home provided the care team visit several times each day, monitor all medication and change it appropriately, and advise the family on fluid intake. Useful medications include the following:

(1) hyoscine butylbromide for colic, given SC as required, every four hours regularly, or, preferably, by syringe-driver. Transdermal patches of hyoscine hydrobromide are not so useful in this condition but may be tried.
(2) opioids, which are seldom needed and are, in any case, not likely to help in the longterm because of the constipation they produce.
(3) a faecal softener (Docusate or lactulose if fluid can be taken) in a dose high enough to make bowel contents fluid so as to negotiate obstructed loops of bowel. (*On no account can a peristaltic stimulant be used.*)
(4) cyclizine 50 milligram three times a day or 150 milligram over 24 hours via a syringe-driver to reduce nausea. Rarely do any other antiemetics have any effect and reliance on them is, in any case, illogical when there is obstruction.
(5) as much fluid as the patient can take—but only in the form of crushed ice cubes, sips of iced drinks, and ice lollipops to suck. Until the bowels move well, no solids must be taken or permitted.
(6) scrupulous oral hygiene.

This regimen has been tested and validated worldwide in palliative care units but is contrary to all that doctors have been taught—'drip and suck' for every case. Within a day or two the obstruction passes off, though admittedly whatever is done it will likely recur, and the patient will have been well cared for at home rather than in a strange, intimidating hospital ward. These patients do *not* develop electrolyte imbalance, nor will they complain of dehydration, but only of dry mouth, thirst, and halitosis.

LYMPHANGITIS CARCINOMATOSIS

Most common in women with carcinoma of breast, this is not easy to diagnose. At first increasing dyspnoea may be thought of as infection or, in an older patient, as cardiac failure and treated accordingly. Often the characteristic widespread crepitations and changed character of the breath sounds are late signs, and even then radiological clues may not be helpful. In some cases early diagnosis is based more on suspicion than on hard objective data or on the presence of a persistent non-productive cough. As it progresses relentlessly, dyspnoea becomes totally disabling and frightening. Inevitably doctors prescribe antibiotics, diuretics, bronchodilators, neubulizers, and so on but mainly to little avail.

Treatment

1. Chemotherapy in early cases because the cause is often a sensitive tumour. This may prove challenging for the family doctor who wants to do what is best for his patient but may feel that by now 'active' treatment is inappropriate and find it difficult to support the recommendation to start or continue with chemotherapy.
2. Steroids, with the opioids, are the only drugs likely to help in any way. Unless there are major contraindications they should be prescribed and maintained as long as the patient can take them as prednisolone 10 milligram three times a day or dexamethasone 4 milligram each morning.
3. Opioids to reduce tachypnoea, but the benefit will not be as great as in 'simple' bronchogenic carcinoma.
4. In the final weeks, the opioids and skilled tranquillizing. These are essential, along with everything possible being done to give the frightened patient a sense of safety.

NAUSEA AND VOMITING

Both symptoms are common in malignant disease and can often prove much more difficult to palliate than pain and many other symptoms. One problem is that often no one single cause can be identified, but this should not stop the family doctor searching for one.

It is worth remembering that nausea is usually more distressing than vomiting. Many patients, though not happy about it, may come to accept an occasional vomit if, between each event, they are not nauseated and can eat reasonably well. Much more distressing for patients and relatives is persistent nausea, even when there is no vomiting.

Causes

1. *Metabolic:* hyper- or hypo-natraemia, hypercalcaemia, uraemia.
2. *Drug-induced:* though usually wrongly implicated, the opioids can produce nausea but only in their first few days of use, when the dose is raised considerably and particularly when too high an initial dose is prescribed (not following the guidelines outlined in this book). Most other medications can

produce nausea in these patients, particularly when renal function is compromised, and each must be suspected and the need for them re-examined. Chemotherapy is a very common cause but not likely to be relevant in the patient at home under the care of the primary care team.

3. *Intestinal obstruction:* The features of this are well known but sometimes forgotten is gastric outlet obstruction. Here the patient only experiences nausea for a few minutes immediately before vomiting, after which he feels so much better than it may feel safe to eat again. This classic description should be enquired about in every case. When the obstruction is high, there is initially as much vomiting as nausea, the vomit usually being bilious rather than faecal, with little if any pain in attacks of subacute obstruction. When the obstruction is lower, often in the colon, there may be little nausea but frequent faecal vomiting, visible peristalsis etc.

4. *Raised intracranial pressure:* will be suggested when the vomiting (rather than any nausea which is usually absent) is a regular early morning occurrence, accompanied by such other features as morning headache, focal neurological signs, and possibly personality change. Usually one can confirm the suspicion by finding papilloedema.

5. *Chronic constipation:* so common in these patients, particularly when taking opioids, can undoubtedly cause nausea and vomiting even when there is not frank intestinal obstruction. Some palliative medicine specialists would go so far as to suggest that this is the commonest cause of nausea and vomiting.

6. *Anxiety state:* particularly if associated with poorly controlled physical symptoms or unaddressed fears.

Management

1. Try to identify the cause and treat appropriately. Much easier said than done, but do not rush into prescribing antiemetics empirically.

2. For drug-induced nausea, use haloperidol 0.5 milligram three times a day or 1.5 milligram daily orally, by injection or subcutaneously via a syringe-driver, remembering the long half-life of this drug and its tendency to sedate the patient.

3. For subacute obstruction (but not gastric outlet obstruction), try cyclizine 50 milligram three times a day orally or by injection or 150–200 milligram per day subcutaneously via a syringe-driver.

4. For gastric outlet obstruction, check with specialist colleagues whether further chemotherapy is appropriate or radiotherapy for glands in the porta hepatis, and in the meantime prescribe a prokinetic such as metoclopramide 10 milligram three or four times a day, or domperidone in the same doses for the older patients, or oral cisapride 10 milligram three times a day. Occasionally the best thing to give is high-dose metoclopramide (60–120 milligram per day) subcutaneously via a syringe-driver until the symptom comes under control. Provided the patient is not on any other drug capable of

producing extra pyraminal effects, this high dose of metoclopramide is safe. In the patient still reasonably well, a gastroenterostomy or percutaneous jejunostomy should be considered, drastic as this may sound.

5. When all else fails, one can either prescribe a drug from another group of antiemetics, (i.e. phenothiazines, butyrophenones or prokinetics, depending on what has already been tried) *or* give empirical dexamethasone, starting with 8 milligram each morning for 2 days, reducing by 2 milligram every 2 or 3 days. This sometimes helps when there are no specific indications such as cerebral oedema, hypercalcaemia, or grossly elevated liver function tests (LFTs).

6. Admit to hospital or palliative care unit. As so often in general practice, it is sometimes helpful to take the patient out of their present environment into one of high professional presence and confidence, whether or not they are then given IV fluids, have further X-rays, or ultrasound scans etc.

NIGHTSWEATS

These are more common than many people appreciate. The patient is uncomfortable and embarrassed because of the extra work falling on relatives and often, secretly, wonders if he has an infectious condition such as tuberculosis or AIDS about which no one has dared to speak. The extra work for relatives can soon lead to a request for readmission to hospital.

Causes

(1) hepatic metastases (whatever the primary malignancy);
(2) infection, usually chronic such as tuberculosis, opportunistic infection in AIDS, and sarcoidosis.

Management

1. Search for, and treat appropriately, any infection.
2. Hepatic metastases:

   (a) when the patient is so ill that death is expected at any time, the answer is in skilled nursing—frequent sponging, application of soothing talcum powder, light bedding, and a nearby fan;

   (b) when liver function tests show rapid, relentless deterioration, worsening every week or so, give dexamethasone 4–6 milligram each morning, reducing to a maintenance of 2–4 milligram when sweating diminishes;

   (c) when LTFs are not rapidly deteriorating and the patient is otherwise relatively well, the only major symptom being this hyperhidrosis, give:

      (i) cimetidine 400 milligram twice a day (or at night only if sweating is only troublesome at night) or (ii) ranitidine 150 milligram twice a day or

(iii) indomethacin 25 milligram three times a day or a sustained release formulation.

Good results will be obtained within days in the majority of patients and the drug should then be continued at that same dose.

OEDEMA

Types of oedema

1. Lymphoedema, whether in arm or leg, can nowadays be reduced quite dramatically by the modern compression bandage technique familiar to most physiotherapists. On the other hand, if there is one nearby, the patient can be referred to a Lymphoedema Clinic. The earlier such patients are treated, the better. There is now no place for Flowtron or Jobst pumps.
2. Bilateral upper limb oedema may be lymphoedema but is more usually a feature of superior vena caval obstruction (SVCO), the management of which is described on p. 71.
3. Unilateral leg oedema may be caused by a deep vein thrombosis (DVT), lymphoedema, or venous obstruction at the level of the internal iliac veins as a result of tumour or nodes.

   In an otherwise relatively well patient, anticoagulants may be justified for DVT but the family doctor, as always, must pause and think before instituting anticoagulants or referring the patient to hospital for heparinization and later warfarin. What will the patient feel about readmission at this time in his life, how easy will it be to monitor his anticoagulant regimen on discharge, will there be increased dangers of bleeding from his tumour (e.g. in bladder or stomach)? Do the potential dangers of pulmonary emboli and infarction at this late stage in life outweigh the drawbacks mentioned?

   Venous obstruction is not reversible but may be improved with pelvic irradiation, unless the area has already had full-dose irradiation, in which case the doctor might care to prescribe dexamethasone 6–8 milligram each morning (later reducing to as low a dose as possible) to reduce tumour and nodal bulk.
4. Bilateral leg oedema, unless of cardiac origin (in which case there would be the many other signs of cardiac failure) will always be found to follow:

   (a) pelvic obstruction from tumour and/or nodes
   (b) inferior vena caval obstruction from para-aortic/para-inferior vena caval nodes possibly already demonstrated on ultrasound scan, computerised tomography (CT), or magnetic resonance imaging (MRI)
   (c) hypoalbuminaemia from liver failure.

In the latter case, the diagnosis will soon be confirmed as the oedema rapidly spreads up from the legs to the perineum (in the male producing penile and scrotal oedema) and over the trunk, always soft and easily pitted on the slightest pressure.

There are few therapeutic options. Elevating the legs modestly reduces the leg oedema whilst worsening that around sacrum and perineum. Rarely if ever is an albumin infusion justified. Diuretics are effective (provided the patient is catheterized to save frequent toileting) but soon the patient is exhausted and reluctant to have to take potassium supplements in addition to all the other medication. If it is decided to use them, if only to reduce modestly the oedema bulk, the preferable drug is frusemide 40–120 milligram daily.

IVC obstruction or hyperalbuminaemic oedema should be regarded as events heralding the final weeks and days of life, and the relatives be so advised.

PERICARDIAL EFFUSION

Fortunately this is a rare condition so far as domiciliary care is concerned. Little need be said about it here except to list the principal causes and suggest management for general practice.

Causes

1. Myocardial infarction
2. Pericarditis (pyogenic, viral, and tuberculous)
3. Malignancy spreading from a neighbouring tumour or mediastinal nodes
4. Metastatic from a distant malignancy.

The symptoms and signs are well known—increasing dyspnoea (sometimes very acute and becoming disabling within hours), muffled heart sound, cardiac tamponade and failure.

Unless the patient is expected to die within a day or two from whatever is the underlying disease, admission to hospital is essential for paracentesis and, if the general condition merits it, the creation of a pericardial window.

If it is decided to keep the patient at home, regarding the pericardial effusion as the terminal event, the patient will require heavy sedation with subcutaneous diamorphine and either diazepam or midazolam, preferably via a syringe-driver to eradicate all panic and restlessness.

PLEURAL EFFUSION

It is sometimes difficult for a family doctor to know how he should manage a terminally ill patient with a pleural effusion. Always assuming the underlying pathology is known, the guidelines are given below.

1. If it is accumulating rapidly, then arrangements should be made for readmission to a familiar ward of unit for elective drainage.
2. If it is diagnosed coincidentally in a patient with no respiratory symptoms whatsoever, it need not be drained but its progress regularly monitored. The patient should certainly not be automatically admitted somewhere with the promise made to patient and relatives that it will be drained.
3. If it is due to mesothelioma it should only be drained as a last resort because of the likelihood of tumour seedlings growing in the needle tract, producing exquisitely tender nodules.
4. If it keeps recurring, the patient should be offered pleurodesis with an agent such as C-parvum, tetracycline, or bleomycin. This will be done in hospital but the patient needs to be prepared by the family doctor explaining the reasons for it, the outlines of the procedure, and the discomfort which inevitably follows for several hours.

It is worth remembering that pleural effusion carries a poor prognosis for almost all malignancies except breast carcinoma patients who may survive with it for many months or even beyond a year.

PRURITUS

Though not common, this symptom can be very distressing to the patient and leave the lay carers at home feeling helpless. It is most usually a feature of biliary obstruction but can also occur in Hodgkin's lymphoma, myeloma, carcinoid syndrome, and macroglobulinaemia.

Management

1. Nursing measures can help to keep the skin cool and lessen perspiration, both of which reduce the itch threshold.
2. Biliary stenting is more effective than any other measure and should be considered for all except the most terminally ill. Usually all jaundice clears, but even if only modestly reduced the pruritus will disappear.
3. Topical measures include calamine lotion, crotamaton cream (with or without steroid), and even the old-fashioned remedy of sodium bicarbonate solution dabbed on the skin, as required, by the patient (one dessertspoon of powder dissolved in a cup of water).
4. Cholestyramine is the drug of first choice, particularly in biliary obstruction, if the patient can tolerate the taste (it should be remembered that cholestyramine worsens steatorrhoea).
5. H_1 receptor blockers and phenothiazines should be tried if cholestyramine fails, but sedation is often unacceptable.

6. A sedative at night is almost always required, the preferable one being tri-meprazine tartrate (Vallergan).
7. H_2 receptor blocker (cimetidine) occasionally helps
8. Rifampicin is likely to help in primary biliary cirrhosis but not in other conditions.

SORE MOUTH

Anything which makes eating painful or difficult is worth treating, as much for the caring relatives who feel that feeding the patient is all that is left to them, as for the patient himself.

Causes

1. Oral candidiasis, present in 60—75 per cent of patients but often missed by doctors who do not always look for it, and nurses who expect to see the classical white plaques rather than equally common red, spongy mucosa and angular stomatitis in denture-wearers;
2. Aphthous ulcers, less common than candidiasis but distressingly painful;
3. Post-chemotherapy stomatitis.

Management

Foods and fluids are usually preferred very cold rather than hot, with semisolids preferable to either fluids or solids.

1. Candidiasis must be taken seriously and treated thoroughly. Most cases will respond to nystatin suspension 1 ml four times a day, provided dentures are taken out and soaked overnight in chlorine-releasing solution (if non-metal) or brushed with povidone—iodine solution (metal dentures). After mouth-rinsing with nystatin, it should be swallowed to prevent candida-oesophagitis and the treatment continued for the rest of the life of these terminally ill patients we are describing. If symptoms and signs of candida persist, it should first be checked whether the above routine has been followed faith-fully. Usually it has not. If it has, the doctor can then give either 2 per cent miconazole gel (or ketoconazole capsules 200 milligram daily) or, preferable but five times the price of nystatin, fluconazole 50 milligram daily for one week.
2. Aphthous ulcers respond to tetracycline suspension mouthwash (10 ml rinse for 2 minutes, then swallowed, every 6 hours) or hydrocortisone pellets 2.5 milligram four times a day sucked as close to the ulcer as possible, or Aschurt's solution (betamethasone) 5—10 ml every 4 hours. This excellent preparation must be prepared freshly for each patient by the pharmacist.

Ulcers of viral (herpetic) origin seen particularly in AIDS patients respond to acyclovir orally 200 milligram every 4 hours for 5 days.
3. Post-chemotherapy stomatitis will eventually clear up spontaneously but the mouth can be made comfortable with:

(a) benzydamine mouthwash (Diflam)
(b) choline salicylate gel (Bonjela)
(c) 0.1 per cent hexetidine (Oraldene)
(d) Aschurt's solution.

Rarely, because of the risk of aspiration due to the profound numbness, lignocaine gel may be used.
4. Xerostomia is a frequent problem even when not assciated with infection and ulceration. Its principal causes are the drugs being taken, mouth breathing, inadequate fluid intake, and inadequate mouthcare. Contrary to what might be expected, xerostomia may persist even after intravenous rehydration. It can be helped by:

(a) sucking thin slices of tinned rather than fresh pineapple
(b) sugarless chewing gum or hydrophilic chewing gum
(c) sucking ice cubes or effervescent vitamin C tablets
(d) artificial saliva.

STEROIDS IN PALLIATIVE CARE

Corticosteroids have many uses in palliative care and at times their benefits can be quite remarkable. However, they are not panaceas, nor are they free of unwanted effects so the same care must be exercised in their use in the terminally ill as at any other time.

The following rules apply to their use in these patients.

1. So far as is possible, prescribe them for specific rather than non-specific indications.
2. Prescribe them for as short a time as possible, aiming to bring the dose down to the lowest possible as speedily as possible.
3. If possible, do not prescribe them for a patient also on NSAIDs, so increasing the likelihood of active peptic ulceration and bleeding up to 15-fold.
4. Do not prescribe them for a patient known to have a dormant infection such as tuberculosis.
5. Ensure they are taken as early in the day as possible and when high doses are needed, certainly not after mid-afternoon to avoid sleep disturbance.
6. Change from dexamethasone to prednisolone when longterm use is envisaged and always by one month (dexamethasone 1 milligram equals prednisolone 7 milligram).
7. Be on the alert for the development of adverse effects.

Specific indications

- Raised intracranial pressure from cerebral oedema (a clinical response may be seen within 24 to 48 hours)
- spinal cord compression
- superior vena caval obstruction
- extrinsic nerve/nerve root compression.

(In each case, especially number 4, a clinical response may be seen within days.)

Dexamethasone dose regimen

1. emergency: 16 milligram per day (intramuscular or oral), reducing by 2 milligram per day to a maintenance dose of 8 milligram per day;
2. maintenance: 8 milligram per day in divided doses reduced as soon as possible by 2 milligram every 3 or 4 days to 2–4 milligram each morning.

Non-specific indications

1. *Anorexia*: The appetite stimulant effect of the steroids seldom lasts beyond 3 weeks. It is easiest to prescribe prednisolone as already described. A more prolonged effect, at vastly greater expense, can be achieved with progestogen megestrol acetate (Megace) 160–480 milligram per day for not less than one month, preferably at the higher dose.
2. *Nausea and/or sweating associated with hepatic metastases*: Here the above maintenance dexamethasone regimen is used. (see 'Nightsweats' p. 54)

Principal adverse effects likely to be seen in palliative care

1. *Neuropsychiatric problems*: The commonest cause is excitability and euphoria bordering on hypomania. If the steroid cannot be reduced, the patient will need chlorpromazine 25–100 milligram three times a day, though doses as high as 1 g per day have been needed. Less common than hypomania but frequently seen are agitated anxiety states, profound depression, or frank psychosis with hallucinations and delusions, almost all necessitating reducing or even cessation of the steroids, occasionally hospital/hospice admission.
2. *Insomnia*: This is very common, almost the norm, and usually results from the patient not being instructed to take the dexamethasone early in the day to mimic the physiological pattern. Rarely is a sedative required if the dosage times are attended to.
3. *Infection*: Even when dormant infection is not activated, most patients develop frank candidiasis in mouth and oesophagus, others inguinal and skin infections, and many women have clinical candida vulvovaginitis.

4. *Voracious appetite*: Desirable as an improved appetite may be, it can become so uncontrolled that patients put on excessive weight just when they are less active and ambulant, even before Cushingoid features develop. It soon becomes embarrassing, particularly to women who have enjoyed slim figures and now hate their altered body image.

5. *Cushingoid features*: This is dose- and time-related. On high doses the syndrome appears early but even on doses as low as dexamethasone 2 milligram or prednisolone 15 milligram daily over many weeks the Cushingoid features become gross. Women in particular are understandably upset by this and the added effects of striae and telangiectasia.

6. *Diabetes mellitus*: This occurs in 5–10 per cent of these patients and may present as subacute diabetic coma, easily mistaken for the terminal phase. Hypoglycaemic agents are rarely required if the dose of steroid is carefully reduced.

7. *Demineralization*: Progressive osteoporosis of the cervical thoracic spine leads to both kyphoscoliosis and low-grade pain across the neck and shoulders, easily attributed to metastases but actually iatrogenic.

8. *Myopathy*: Often said to be 'proximal' myopathy, it is indeed most seen in shoulder and pelvic girdle muscles but can also be observed in such muscles as the diaphragm, producing progressive dyspnoea.

9. *Burning perineal pain*: This is rare and appears only to develop when high-dose dexamethasone (up to 100 milligram) is given IV.

10. *Avascular necrosis of the femoral head*: This is reported but probably uncommon.

11. *Peptic ulceration*: Doubts exist whether corticosteroids alone can lead to ulceration. There is no good evidence that H_2 antagonists are needed or useful as prophylactics. On the other hand, taking a corticosteroid along with any NSAID increases the risk of peptic ulceration and bleeding by a factor of 10 to 15.

SUPERIOR VENA CAVAL OBSTRUCTION (SVCO)

Though rarely seen by the family doctor, this complication of several malignancies must be remembered because it can produce extreme distress, yet is readily responsive to palliative treatment.

The patient will probably have been known to have a bronchogenic carcinoma, one of the reticuloses, or some other cause of hilar/mediastinal adenopathy which then compresses the superior vena cava. The symptoms are of steadily, often rapidly, increasing dyspnoea, eventually so disabling that no activity is possible. The signs are diagnostic—pouches of infraorbital oedema, elevated jugular venous pressure (JVP), dilated collateral vessels coursing across the anterior chest wall, and a striking appearance of someone bloated from the chest upwards, struggling to breathe on minimal exertion.

Management

1. Where there are still theraputic options, the underlying disease should continue to be targeted and treated in the hope that that will reduce the adneopathy and so relieve the SVCO.
2. If radiotherapy can be given within days, this should be arranged as a matter of urgency, referring the patient *directly* to a radiotherapy unit.
3. For immediate relief, whether or not radio- or chemotherapy are being offered, the patient can be given dexamethasone:

   (a) as an emergency: intramuscular 16 milligram reducing by 4 milligram per day, always given before 2pm
   (b) as maintenence: 8 milligram per day, reducing gradually to 2 milligram per day, again taken before 2pm.

WEAKNESS AND LETHARGY

These symptoms are inevitable in all patients with far-advanced disease, whether cardiac, respiratory, malignant, or degenerative. Understandable as this is to doctors and nurses, few patients ever expect to become so weak and tired and often describe these symptoms as the most trying and depressing features of their illness: 'I can accept the discomfort and the poor appetite, but I hate feeling so weak and having to have so much done for me!'. Relatives often plead with the doctor to restore energy, urging him to consider tonics, blood transfusion, or total parenteral nutrition, apparently unable to accept that frailty and dependency are inseparable from chronic dying.

Having said that, the doctor is still obliged to look for treatable causes of the weakness and lethargy.

1. Boredom is common in these patients particularly when pain and other symptoms have been well palliated, leaving the patient free to enjoy what life is left but no one has sought means to break his boredom. *This is where a day hospice is invaluable.* If there is not one nearby an occupational therapist should be called in, adjustment made to the timing of friends' visits, and advice and suggestions given about *creative* activities (and not just time-filling tasks). Even the frail can do craftwork, sort stamps, catalogue recipes and addresses, draw, paint, model, write, make a tape or video for the family—provided it reinforces their usefulness.
2. Excessive sedation or analgesia can be reduced.
3. Depression must be considered and treated as suggested on p. 40.
4. Metabolic causes such as hypercalcaemia, hypokalaemia, and hyponatraemia should be treated.
5. Adrenal failiure, unless a terminal event, is worth treating. It may follow hypophysectomy, adrenalectomy, and aminoglutethimide therapy, especially

if the patient has for some reason failed to take steroid replacements, or developed an infection.

As always, any investigation should only be done if the result might lead to treatment with a worthwhile result in terms of the quality of life for the patient, not because it will help the doctor or nurse to feel better!

3 Diet

Here we must look at two separate issues; the significance of diet to the patient and relatives, and the advice the doctor can give to help them. It is easy for a doctor to dismiss the subject as unimportant by the time a patient has advanced illness but this will rarely, if ever, be how the relatives view the subject of diet. If the doctor fails to address the question of diet, patients and their carers will turn elsewhere or come to their own solutions which may well be inappropriate or even harmful.

THE LAYMAN'S VIEW

It would be a bold newspaper editor or magazine proprietor who thought he could attract readers without a section in his publication on diet or menus. From our earliest days we are given to understand that much depends on what and how we eat. Some facts are well proven, others but passing fads and fancies with little evidence to support them. Every day our patients are bombarded by claims of manufacturers and advertisers anxious to boost their sales, with few of their readers qualified to refute quasiscientific claims. Some of these popular notions, listed here, true and false, need to be remembered by those caring for the dying.

1. Without food we die (and the corollary, if we keep up a good nutritional intake we live). This is true but only up to a point. That point is when the patient has reached the stage of far-advanced malignancy, AIDS, or other chronic disease by which time they are cachectic and liver function is such that the body cannot any longer adequately metabolize or utilize its food intake. Defining that point is difficult. Many cancer patients who are still able to benefit from chemotherapy do respond to well-planned dietary intake, sometimes in the form of total parenteral nutrition (TPN). In this book we are looking at the care and needs of people beyond that stage. It requires considerable skill and patience to explain to relatives when the patient is no longer likely to benefit. They have to be told that a reduced intake or the stopping of TPN is not meant to shorten life, nor is it evidence of professional indifference or callousness; rather, it is a recognition that that life is coming to an end because of the underlying pathology, not because of medically-sanctioned starvation.

2. Certain foods have specific healing or therapeutic qualities. Many people are convinced that megadose vitamins or regular iron intake can work miracles in delaying the inevitable. Even doctors persist in urging patients to take oral iron preparations when their adverse gastrointestinal effects are obvious and upsetting, and even when their patient has to have a red cell concentrate infusion every four weeks—evidence if any was needed that the iron is not helping. Other relatives, convinced since childhood that health depends on daily milk, force the patient to drink it or give it in 'invalid' foods, not acknowledging his nausea or the inevitable constipation.

3. All medically recommended diets are complicated. To some extent this belief is well founded. All doctors come to learn how patients find diabetic diets difficult to understand. Many patients only manage to adhere to them because they do so blindly with little understanding of their basis. For example, they over-simplify the subject of believing that all that matters is that sugar is restricted. Similarly, patients find the protein restriction diet for renal failure difficult, partly because they do not understand the difference between carbohydrate, fat, and protein and do not know which foods contain which. When the patient has life-threatening or terminal disease, he assumes that the diet he must follow is complicated beyond his understanding. Rather than fail the patient, the carers ask for exact details of what must be eaten, in what quantities, and when, as if life itself depended on it. The simple advice to 'give him what he fancies when he wants it' can frighten them by its stark simplicity. It sounds too simple to be true. They turn elsewhere for help—to friends and neighbours, to alternative healers, and to complete charlatans, only to be disappointed and then feel a failure.

4. Preparing and serving good meals is the wife's duty to the end. This is not a misconception but a reflection of this sense of helplessness in the face of death. Most wives see their final role as the continuing provider of nourishment for the husband or dying child. There is little else they feel qualified to do but cook and offer 'good' meals, each meant to keep him alive a little longer, each a social event as in happier days. When the patient will not eat, they see it not as a feature of his decline but as a mark of their failure, of their choice of food, or of their cooking and its presentation.

Each of these notions must be borne in mind by the doctor. He can ignore them or address them. In the months and years to come relatives will often look back and recount how the doctor helped them with dietary problems or ignored their needs and let the patient die. If his advice was complicated, they may take fright and request admission so that the diet can become the responsibility of the experts—the hospital doctors, nurses and dieticians. If the general practitioner encourages them to slacken some of the previous dietary rules on which the patient's life was said to depend, he may be seen as hastening the death. Many examples come to mind. The insulin-dependent diabetic is in the final weeks of life, scarcely able to eat and so requiring little if any insulin, his blood sugar estimations confirming this. The family (but seldom the patient) may be aghast at this advice to let him have what he fancies! The relative of a patient who has been on iron for years cannot understand how life can go on without it. The husband of a longterm cardiac patient is puzzled by the doctor permitting a little salt.

DIETARY GUIDELINES

When a patient is in the final weeks of life, irrespective of his pathology, the following will be noticed.

1. He will vary from day to day in what he wants, how much he will take, and when he takes it. Some days he will eat well, but the following day may eat nothing. On some days, he will eat one good meal and refuse all others. This is quite normal but needs to be explained.
2. He will usually eat more in the morning than at midday, and almost nothing in the evening. This may be the opposite of his lifelong habit of a simple breakfast, a light lunch and a hearty evening meal with the family. Now breakfast may be two courses, even a cooked breakfast, but by evening he may need much persuasion to take even a small plate of soup.
3. The nearer the patient is to death, the more he will prefer all intake to be either very hot or icy cold. Drinks will be sipped almost too hot to take or, particularly in the week or so before he dies, he will only take drinks straight from the refrigerator, regularly topped up with ice. Ice cream, sorbet, iced yogurt, and cold custard may never have been enjoyed before in his life but now he will happily take one or other every few hours, sometimes asking for them in the middle of the night. This, again, is quite normal but should be explained.
4. The body seems to know what food it can digest. This is certainly not true throughout life but is a feature of end-stage disease. There is little need to advise the nauseated patient to abstain from fries and fat-containing foods. Even a man who has always enjoyed large helpings will now appreciate dainty servings. These patients do not need to be asked about flavourings and spices but will instinctively not take highly-seasoned foods. High roughage food, to be commended when the patient is well, will now be unacceptable as will almost all fancy or 'luxury' food.
5. The dying person rarely appreciates how much fluid his body needs. The lay person cannot be expected to understand how much water is lost through respiration and sweating but will usually be conscious of how much they lose in vomiting and diarrhoea.

All these features can and should be explained to patients and relatives. It can be immensely reassuring to a person to know that they are not unusual in enjoying larger breakfasts than before, or in wanting foods they may scarcely have taken since childhood such as ice cream, blancmange, jelly, custard, and the like.

When the explanation is given to the patient and carers *together* it relieves the tension which often exists when carers are forcing food on the patient only to have it rejected, and also strengthens the arm of the carer who is encouraging a better fluid intake. Even better when doctor and community nurse speak with one voice.

Special requirements

Liquidized diet for oesophageal carcinoma patients

Most hospitals and hospices have a Celestin or Atkinson tube to show patients what size of lumen exists for their intake. Usually they are surprised at how large it is but, at the same time, can be shown the ease with which it will block if white bread is taken or he tries to eat lumps of meat from a casserole! Large group practices would be well advised to have such a tube available for demonstration purposes.

The need for soda water (or other aerated drink) to be taken before and throughout each meal cannot be over-stressed, whether or not the patient has an oesophageal tube *in situ*. Another tip is to take a small drink of honey in warm water before the meal to lubricate the tube.

It is not sufficient merely to prohibit white bread. Patients need to be warned against sandwiches, scones, buns, dry biscuits, and the like, but reminded that they can take toast buttered when it is cold. They need to be told the maximum size of any lumps of food which can be swallowed, and repeatedly told to take 'little and often' whether liquidized or needing a spoon. Advice usually readily understood is, 'No knives or forks from now, only food you would normally take on a spoon'.

High-fluid intake

Relatives should be advised to have an assortment of flavoured drinks in the refrigerator, including the athlete's favourite—equal parts of milk (whole or part-skimmed) and soda water. In addition they should be encouraged to make 'lollipops' in the freezer and to have polythene bags of ice cubes ready to be crushed for sucking. Most will already know that to flavour them they need about equal parts of flavoured juice and water. If they can afford it, they should have some cubes of their favourite tipple such as sherry, port or dilute Drambuie or Cherry Brandy. They soon come to appreciate that patients take in much more fluid (without vomiting) when it comes from sucking crushed ice and that by observing the colour and volume of urine they can judge whether the intake (and renal function) is satisfactory.

Laxative foods

Constipation and advanced disease go hand in hand. With opioids, even the weak ones, constipation is inevitable and rarely will it be prevented or treatable by diet alone. This is frequently forgotten by doctors. Nevertheless, it is useful to advise on appropriate foods, and to list the inappropriate ones if it will reduce the need for laxatives when so many other medications must be taken.

Most patients believe that all breakfast cereals have equal value as fibre intake. They may know that bran products 'keep you regular' but not appreciate that the favourite corn and rice products are constipating! The doctor may be inclined to recommend the addition of bran to porridge and soup, but these more seriously ill patients can rarely tolerate it and most abhor the inevitable flatulence and abdominal distension. They often regard all fruit as laxative, not appreciating that raw apples are constipating because of the pectin content, but stewed or baked apples are laxative because of the sugar or honey added. Some think of bananas as useful laxatives but they are not, though plums, raspberries, currants and tomatoes certainly are.

Sooner or later the doctor will have to review the milk consumption, taken as straight milk or as chocolate drinks, custard, blancmange, milk jelly etc. The nutritional value is unquestioned but the constipating effect has to be considered. Incidentally, there is no need to ration the milk intake for patients with malignant hypercalcaemia.

One final point. The popular laxative *lactulose* is an osmotic laxative, its effect being dependent on a high fluid intake. When this cannot be guaranteed, an alternative laxative must be prescribed.

Previous dietary practice

The diabetic will have to be as careful as ever whilst still eating well, but rarely does the same care need to be exercised when intake falls almost to nil. This will be obvious to the doctor but appear very hazardous to the carers as already explained.

The low protein diet of the renal patient is a similar problem; again the restrictions may be able to be lifted in the final weeks of life.

The gluten-free diet of the coeliac will have to be maintained until very near the end of life if he is not to suffer bulky stools bordering on diarrhoea.

The 'high iron content' diet so beloved of the chronic anaemic patient may never have been much respected by the doctor, but some patients are convinced they have only survived so long because of the liver, red meats, spinach, and milk! They are usually persuaded that the diet is no longer proving its worth when the doctor reports how low the haemoglobin level has become on the diet. If he is wise he will not then prescribe oral iron preparations (with the resultant bowel effects) but consider whether a transfusion of red cell concentrate might help the patient. This decision is not easy. The patient's lethargy, weakness, and confusion may be secondary to iron deficiency anaemia but are equally likely to be the result of the advancing malignancy or chronic infection. It can be disheartening to a patient to be admitted for blood transfusion and to be told after it how rich his blood has become, yet still feel as tired as he was before it. Some, like the author, would say that dyspnoea and angina are the only good indications for blood transfusion in patients with far-advanced disease, in particular malignancy.

In summary, dietary advice for these patients and their caring families is, of necessity, simple, unsophisticated, and apparently common sense, so obvious that it need hardly be mentioned, but it does need to be discussed.

The long-held notions and increasing apprehensions and frustration of patients and families must be addressed. If not, the doctor will find the carer looking elsewhere for guidance, the patient feeling a nuisance or a burden, and the relatives soon asking for him to be admitted, bringing to a premature end the care at home for which everyone had been working.

4 Emergencies in palliative care

It has been said that there are two types of doctor, the proactive and the reactive. Without any doubt, those who practise good palliative care are always proactive. They have to be. They must try to anticipate problems and, with their nursing colleagues, plan accordingly. Undoubtedly the same can be said for nurses though, because of the manner in which they are brought in to share in the care of such patients, they must often feel that the reactive role is given to them. However, not everything can be anticipated. Crises do occur and can constitute genuine emergencies in palliative care. This chapter deals with such emergencies; it must not be forgotten that, to some extent, they can all be expected to occur often enough for the good doctor to be ready for them with the right drugs in his bag. It is important that the doctor does not automatically send the patient back into hospital where the response may not always be appropriate for the patient with far-advanced disease.

SPINAL CORD COMPRESSION (SCC)

Any patient known to have spinal metastases is a candidate for this, particularly if the metastases are in the mid and lower dorsal spine. The most common primary malignancies are in breast, bronchus, prostate, cervix, and thyroid.

There may be no warning symptoms, but occasionally such a patient will report difficulty in voiding urine. There may be hesitancy, or a poor stream, or retention with overflow. More frequently these features are not spontaneously reported and unless routinely asked about may go unnoticed by the doctor.

The other warning symptom which should be remembered and asked about is slight weakness or numbness in one or both legs. The patient may report only that he has felt weaker or been unsteady on his legs, but both the patient and family often attribute this to his being in bed so much.

Paralysis, developing very suddenly with no accompanying pain, is most likely due to a vascular accident but the family doctor would be advised to manage the case as he would if metastatic compression was suspected.

The emergency itself may present as a sudden bilateral nerve root pain radiating from the affected area but more usually it is silent, painless. Acute urinary retention develops, accompanied by varying degrees of weakness or paralysis, dysaesthesia or total anaesthesia, with diminution or loss of reflexes and inability to stand or walk. Examination confirms the neurological features and may also show hypoaesthesia immediately below the affected dermatome.

Management

1. This is a genuine emergency requiring immediate action. If diagnosed within 18—24 hours of it happening, neurosurgical decompression may be effective but some neurosurgeons will not operate on a patient with a bronchogenic carcinoma because of the short prognosis. *Immediate* telephone discussion with a neurosurgeon is essential unless a radiotherapist, alert to the possibility of SCC, has said he can be contacted at any time.
2. If the SCC is over 24 hours old, or if recommended by the neurosurgeon, the patient can sometimes be helped by urgent radiotherapy. Once again, *immediate* action and referral is called for, with hospital admission and either MRI (if available) or a myelogram performed to locate the site of compression.
3. When both options are impossible, high-dose dexamethasone occasionally helps. The initial dose should be 24 milligram in the first 24 hours, followed by 20 milligram, 16 milligram, 12 milligram, and 8 milligram doses on succeeding days. If benefit follows, it will be obvious within 48 hours or the steroid can be discontinued abruptly. Clearly, it is essential to carry a vial of dexamethasone in the doctor's bag for such an emergency (and others described in this and other chapters).
4. The patient should be catheterized, whatever other course of action is followed.

If this tragic complication is discovered too late to reverse, the doctor is faced with the question whether or not the patient, now paraplegic but probably pain-free in the spine, can still be nursed at home. The answer will depend on the availability of nurses, assistance in the house, the ability and availability of relatives, and the home situation. It should be remembered that the mean survival is three months even in the otherwise relatively well cancer patient who becomes paraplegic.

SUPERIOR VENA CAVAL OBSTRUCTION (SVCO)

This complication may occur with any condition producing mediastinal adenopathy, including the reticuloses, bronchogenic, breast, and thyroid carcinomata. Unlike SCC which can develop within hours, superior vena caval obstruction develops over a few weeks, at first scarcely apparent but finally debilitating enough to constitute an emergency. Knowing of the possibility of its development in such patients, it ought to be anticipated and regularly looked for.

Dyspnoea is severe even at rest and particularly at night when it may mimic paroxysmal nocturnal dyspnoea. Colateral veins appear on the anterior chest wall, oedematous bags show under the eyes, giving a characteristic picture; JVP is raised and cyanosis may develop in the advanced stages. The overall picture is of someone bloated and puffy as if holding his breath or straining.

Management

1. If the patient has not had full-dose radiotherapy to the mediastinum, this should be arranged with the radiotherapist *as a matter of urgency.*
2. If no further radiation can be given, or for other reasons the patient cannot be sent to the radiotherapist, the doctor can give high-dose dexamethasone in the same dosage regimen as described above for SCC. Benefit is seen within 48 hours, often within 24 hours. The patient should then be maintained on dexamethasone 2–4 milligram each morning indefinitely.

When successfully treated, the prognosis is that of the underlying malignancy. If treatment is not given, or is unsuccessful, the patient will die a distressing, dyspnoeic, frightening death, usually within a few weeks.

CONVULSIONS

Here we are not considering convulsions as the presenting feature of a space-occupying lesion or cerebrovascular accident (CVA), but at those occurring in a patient already diagnosed as having primary or secondary malignancy in the brain or subsequent to neurosurgery. Ten per cent of all terminally ill cancer patients have one or more fits. The most common secondaries are those originating in bronchogenic carcinomata, particularly small cell tumours, breast, and melanoma. It has to be remembered that the cerebral metastases may not have been suspected or diagnosed when the far-advanced state of the disease was demonstrated. The secondaries may be so small in the case of malignant melanoma that even a brain scan may not show them. The possibility of convulsions should therefore be borne in mind in patients with any of the malignancies mentioned above.

Some would argue that to warn relatives of the possibility of fits could be so frightening that they might not be willing to have the patient at home; better to wait and see if they occur rather than alarm them. The author would suggest otherwise and recommend that, when there is a strong possibility of convulsions (for example, when cerebral metastases have already been demonstrated) many relatives will benefit from being forewarned. Not only can fits be described and the management outlined, but the real possibility of keeping the patient at home in spite of them can be explained and explored. Clearly the subject is a difficult and delicate one, demanding the communication skills so often called for and present in general practice.

Management

1. If the doctor can be on the scene within minutes, the patient can be given IV diazepam (Diazemuls) 10 milligram at the rate of 1 milligram per minute,

or IV midazolam 5–10 milligram, given at the same rate. Perhaps it does not need to be said that diazepam should not be given intramuscularly because it takes more than an hour to achieve adequate plasma levels.

2. When such prompt attendance is impossible, relatives can be left with a supply of rectal diazepam solution (Stesolid) and instructed in how to give 20 milligram at the commencement of a fit. It will be effective in 10–15 minutes and last for 3 hours. (The relatives will need instruction on maintaining an airway, removal of dentures, loosening of tight collars, etc.)

3. As prophylaxis, most patients will be able to take phenytoin so long as they can swallow. When that is impossible, they will need daily intramuscular injections by the community nurse of sodium phenobarbitone 100–200 milligram or the addition of midazolam to the analgesic in the syringe-driver. Alternatively, a specially prepared aqueous solution of phenobarbitone can be given via a syringe-driver.

If raised intracranial pressure producing papilloedema is found on retinoscopy, the difficult question arises of whether or not the dose of dexamethasone should be increased. This should not be an automatic response. It requires most careful consideration.

In the patient already known to have far-advanced malignancy but no proven cerebral metastases, the presence of raised intracranial pressure is highly suggestive of such secondaries. A brain scan would confirm them but almost inevitably there would be delay in getting it done, and the interim the cerebral oedema should be reduced with dexamethasone in a dose of 8 milligram per day (given in divided doses before mid-afternoon so as not to produce disturbed sleep at night), reducing by 2 milligram per day every 3 or 4 days until a maintenance dose of 2 milligram per day is achieved. Should a scan be thought necessary, and always bearing in mind the frailty of such a patient, the existence of one or more metastases would raise the question of whether focal or whole brain irradiation was justified. Rarely will surgical excision of a solitary secondary be appropriate in a patient already so ill, except in the case of cerebellar secondaries when surgical excision is often highly successful. There is no place for chemotherapy for cerebral metastases at this stage of the illness.

The patient already on dexamethasone is a different problem. An increase in the drug from its low maintenance dose to e.g. 8 milligram or even more, is usually justified on the first occasion of fits due to oedema and tumour bulk. Again, attempts should be made to reduce it as quickly as possible.

There comes a stage, however, when it seems inappropriate to boost a dose yet again. Each time it has been done the response will have been noted to be less satisfactory and all the while the general condition has been deteriorating. Dexamethasone is, in one sense, like a life support system—easy to initiate but difficult to withdraw and of diminishing value. One of the necessary skills of a doctor supervising domiciliary palliative care is knowing when enough is enough, and being able to explain and discuss this issue with the relatives, and indeed with the patient if that is possible.

As all are aware, longterm use of dexamethasone is not without its problems—not only of gastrointestinal bleeding, Cushingoid features, skin and capillary fragility, and demineralization of bone, but also of steroid-induced proximal myopathy. The latter is irreversible and makes rising from a chair, and hence the nursing of an already frail patient, even more difficult. Myopathy can also affect the diaphragm producing dyspnoea.

HAEMORRHAGE

Contrary to what most lay people imagine, catastrophic haemorrhage is rare. The author has seen only one in 20 years in this work. Such a statistic is not likely to reassure either patient or relative if someone at home has a haematemesis, haemoptysis, or bladder haemorrhage so obvious in the catheter bag. Preventions is, as always, better than cure and once again the doctor will find himself having to decide whether to admit the patient to hospital. If the patient is still relatively well in spite of advanced disease, admission for emergency blood transfusion is probably justified. If already frail, and possibly bedbound, nothing is to be gained unless the doctor feels the threat of further, possibly fatal, haemorrhage is more than the family can cope with.

Gastric haemorrhage is the most common, often due to gastric carcinoma, oesophageal varices, or following the use of NSAIDs for bone metastases, particularly if a steroid has inadvertently been prescribed concomitantly. The combination of an NSAID and steroid increases the risk of haemorrhage tenfold. There is no evidence that the prophylactic use of an H_2 antagonist reduces this risk.

Massive pulmonary haemorrhage is less commonly seen now that palliative radiotherapy is given in the earlier stages of treatment of bronchogenic carcinoma, but erosion of a major vessel remains a possibility.

Haematuria is very common, almost the norm, in patients with advanced bladder carcinoma and occasionally in those with renal carcinoma, but seldom constitutes an emergency. Much can be done at an earlier stage to reduce it and patients and relatives have hopefully had its cause carefully explained to them.

Management

1. For massive, potentially fatal haemorrhage the immediate priority is to sedate the patient because fear and agitation will only make the situation worse. The doctor should give SC or IV diamorphine 10–20 milligram, though much higher doses will be needed and can safely be given when the patient is already on the drug for analgesia. The rule in that case is to give *not less than* one-sixth of the total daily intake but up to one quarter can be used safely.

2. An alternative is SC/IV midazolam 5−10 milligram if the patient is not already on the drug or one-sixth (up to one-quarter) of the total daily dose in those already on the drug.
3. If the doctor is unlikely to be able to get to the patient quickly enough to give these injections, the family can be given rectal diazepam solution (Stesolid) and instructed to give 20 milligram immediately. If the haemorrhage is a large and potentially fatal one, this is not likely to be effective in time because it requires 10−15 minutes to take effect.

The question whether or not to arrange emergency admission to hospital has been mentioned. Much will depend on the site and magnitude of the haemorrhage, the general condition of the patient, family and primary care resources, and everyone's expectations.

If it looks as though death will occur within an hour or so, transfer to hospital is ill-advised. If it does not occur in the ambulance, it may happen within minutes of arrival in hospital. The family may blame the journey (and the doctor for suggesting it) and almost inevitably the junior hospital staff will react reflexively by setting up an intravenous drip and instituting resuscitation procedures, quite inappropriate in such a patient. If the haemorrhage is smaller but likely to be a warning of more to come, the doctor must decide whether the family (and colleagues) can cope. Provided the patient is heavily sedated and the relatives fully informed of what lies ahead, it may be better to keep the patient at home. If admission is thought preferable, the doctor must make contact with the hospital, fully explain the advanced nature of the patient's illness, and his reasons for requesting admission with the understanding that emergency transfusion and energetic resuscitative measures are not immediately and reflexively started.

It should be remembered that, if the paramedic ambulance crew arrive at the house and find the patient dead or near dead, they will attempt resuscitation by all means available unless (a) a letter is left for them by the doctor instructing that no resuscitation must be attempted or (b) these instructions are conveyed by telephone to ambulance control when the call is made. Regulations do not permit paramedics to exercise discretion in such cases.

ACUTE HYPERCALCAEMIA

Though malignant hypercalcaemia usually develops over days or weeks, it may occasionally present as an emergency. It will present as an acute confusional state but careful history-taking will reveal increasing weakness, polydipsia, and polyuria in the preceding days, all features which may have been accepted as those of the progressive malignancy or cachexia. The suspicion can only be confirmed by biochemical estimation of calcium and albumin to calculate the corrected calcium level (remembering not to leave the tourniquet on when drawing blood).

Management

1. If confusion and agitation are so bad that sedation is necessary whilst awaiting emergency biochemistry tests, it is best to give SC midazolam 2.5–5 milligram, expecting it to tranquillize the patient for 2 hours (larger doses up to 15–20 milligram being needed for someone already on the drug or with a history of longterm benzodiazepine use).
2. Hypercalcaemia cannot usually be treated satisfactorily at home. The patient should be admitted as an emergency for IV saline and pamidronate. Benefit both clinical and biochemical will be apparent within 48–72 hours, after which the patient may be able to return home, possibly on oral bisphosphonates. Normocalcaemia will be maintained for 21–28 days after intravenous bisphosphonates, after which the hypercalcaemia will probably recur. It is therefore important for the family doctor to perform regular calcium and albumin estimations to anticipate and be prepared for future crises. Should hypercalcaemia ever be left untreated at home? The answer is yes in patients so ill and frail that the hypercalcaemia is clearly the final complication and burden for them. Correcting it would not improve the overall quality of life. Left untreated it usually heralds death within a week. What is needed is mild sedation, scrupulous oral hygiene, and good nursing.
3. It is, however, worth remembering that the features of hypercalcaemia so mimic many of those of far-advanced disease that it is not always easy to know how much to attribute to the underlying condition and how much to the hypercalcaemia. Another difficult challenge for the doctor!

The results of appropriate management of hypercalcaemia are often very dramatic and rewarding, the patient apparently being brought back from the brink of death. Ever afterwards the relatives may suspect that any deterioration in the patient's condition is due to a recurrence of the hypercalcaemia, and keep demanding biochemical estimations or hospital admissions, finding it difficult to recognize that the changes are more likely due to progression of the underlying disease.

ACUTE URINARY RETENTION

In addition to the usual cause of benign prostatic hyperplasia in males, retention in the terminally ill may follow the use of tricyclic antidepressants, faecal impaction of the rectum, clot retention even in the catheterized patient, acute urinary infection and, sometimes overlooked, opioid use. Less common, but very important, it may be a presenting feature of spinal cord compression.

Management

Management entails immediate catheterization by the family doctor (who must therefore carry a sterile catheter and anaesthetic gel in his bag). There is no reason why a terminally ill patient should be sent to hospital merely for catheterization, yet that does happen. Having relieved the retention the doctor will attempt to define the cause of it, although hopefully he will be reluctant to take the patient off opioids if they are incriminated, preferring to leave the patient with a regularly lavaged indwelling catheter.

ACUTE PANIC AND PARANOID ATTACKS

It is difficult to conceive of anyone with a fatal illness not sometimes being fearful or apprehensive. Such attacks may occur in the silent stoics as well as the lifelong worriers. Anything can trigger a panic attack—a pain or a newly discovered lump, breathlessness, choking over a crumb, a TV news bulletin, or the arrival of a relative—the list is endless. One has an impression that panic attacks are more common in those who more usually present a façade of calm control.

Management

1. Here we must differentiate between panic and paranoid attacks. The former require a doctor to sit and explore the feelings of the patient before reaching for syringe or prescription pad. The latter require immediate and adequate sedation with haloperidol, intravenously if possible. The initial dose should be 5 milligram, repeated an hour later if paranoid agitation continues, and at 3 or 4 hour intervals until the patient is heavily sedated, after which he must be observed carefully. In the first few days, doses as high as 20–30 milligram per day in single doses may be required, then reduced to a maintenance of 5 milligram in view of this drug's long half-life. The most common mistake is giving too low a starting dose with the result that the patient is drowsy but still conscious enough to be even more suspicious. In many cases urgent hospital or hospice admission is justified for acute paranoia, as much for the sake of the relatives as the patient.
2. Panic attacks are so often due to unventilated fears which are, themselves, based on ignorance or poor understanding of what is happening to them. Time *must* be spent exploring this. It is best to be direct in questioning the patient at these times. Are they frightened of pain in case no one will be able to stop it? Are they scared of fighting for breath, choking over food, bleeding, becoming confused or 'going mad', or (and this can be asked) of death itself?

More often than not a trigger for the attack will be found. The fleck of haemoptysis prompted a fear of dying from bleeding; increasing dyspnoea made the patient think of dying from asphyxia; an episode of forgetfulness or muddledness felt like the features they associate with mental illness or dementia; the sight of an old photograph of a lost loved one brought back memories of his 'awful death' or a death-bed vigil.

'People fear the unknown more than the known.' 'Fears breed on ignorance.' Nowhere are these sayings more true than in the delicate care and support of the dying. Unventilated fears breed panic attacks. The family doctor is in a unique position amongst all the professionals sharing in the care to keep the patient fully informed and to defuse many fears as they arise, long before they erupt as panic.

3. Drugs are but one small part of the response but are usually needed for these attacks. The best for panic is SC or IV midazolam 5—10 milligram, short-acting and markedly amnesogenic. This latter property may be useful but not if a doctor hopes the patient will remember the information and reassurance he gave around the time of the injection! An alternative is IV diazepam (Diazemuls) 5—10 milligram given at the rate of 1 milligram per minute.

4. Patients may benefit from having a small supply of lorazepam tablets 1 milligram for just such a crisis, taking 0.5 milligram or 1 milligram sublingually, but the danger is that they will resort too readily to this rather than getting to the bottom of their fears. This danger is very real and well-recognized by family doctors, who wisely prescribe lorazepam only rarely for other patients.

5. Rarely, a doctor will feel that he needs to put the patient onto a regular, long half-life benzodiazepine such as diazepam once-daily. It should be remembered that a person long dependent on these drugs will require much more than would normally be thought adequate. Similarly, a patient on high-dose opioids will also require proportionately higher dozes of benzodiazepines, phenothiazines, or butyrophenones for whatever reason they are prescribed. It is wrong to assume, as some doctors do, that opioids produce euphoria, but it is correct to believe that the longterm use of them may actually produce dysphoria.

6. It is impossible to calm and reassure a dying patient when all around is tension, activity, and fear. Time spent with the patient will need to be balanced by at least as much time with the relatives whose fears are equally intense, though often for different reasons. Once again the family doctor is in a unique position to help

7. Perhaps it should not need to be said, but the nurses must be kept fully informed of what has been said to the patient and, in particular, what explanations have been given. When one partner in this care is thought to be saying something different from another, the resulting confusion can produce more fear and panic. Five minutes sharing information each morning is never time wasted in good domiciliary care.

PATHOLOGICAL FRACTURES

The ease with which any bone may fracture at the site of a metastasis is well known. There need be no major trauma but merely a change in position, a cough, or a slip off the commode.

Often the site is obvious, as in the clavicle or humerus, but not infrequently a fracture in a femoral neck initially goes unnoticed. The doctor is told of increased pain but no one knows where or why; the opioid is steadily increased but to no avail. Sometimes it is only when the patient is admitted to a palliative care or oncology unit with 'intractable pain' that the shortened externally-rotated leg gives the clue. It cannot be over-stressed that every new pain, every inexplicable need for increased analgesia, must be explored and this demands a careful physical examination.

Management

1. Once again this need not necessitate automatic hospital admission. A fractured clavicle can be treated at home unless it is thought advisable to have the metastasis irradiated. A fracture of the surgical head of humerus can also be managed at home in someone too frail to travel.
2. The priority with a fractured neck of femur or femoral shaft is relief of pain. This is not usually achievable with analgesics alone. Orthopaedic surgery with pinning of a femoral neck, even hip replacement or pin and plating in the shaft, can mean a return home within days and little if any increase in opioids.
3. In the rare case of a bedbound patient with only a few weeks to live sustaining a fracture of the femoral shaft, or being unable to be removed to hospital, the doctor can have the leg sandbagged and inject the fracture site with 10–15 ml of 2 per cent lignocaine. Once the pain has subsided, he can leave a polythene needle or cannula near the site and connect it to a syringe-driver, infusing no more than 20 ml per day of 2 per cent lignocaine. Over the succeeding days, the daily requirement of lignocaine will be found to drop to around 10 ml per day. Thus the patient can be kept remarkably comfortable yet remain at home.

ACUTE INTESTINAL OBSTRUCTION

Acute, or more commonly subacute, intestinal obstruction is relatively common in patients with intraabdominal malignancy arising in pancreas and colon, and occurs in between 40 and 50 per cent of women with carcinoma of ovary.

Though colic may be a feature, it can be totally absent, the pain being more constant in nature, accompanied by nausea, vomiting (not faecal until late-stage), without bowel action but still some flatus, and abdominal distension usually without visible peristalsis. Characteristically, bowel sounds are reduced (so different from the excessive bowel sounds of acute obstruction which possibly led to the original diagnosis) or absent when there is ileus.

Management

Hospital admission need not be the reflex response of the doctor. Nowhere is it more true that each case must be dealt with individually and thoughtfully on its merits.

1. Ovarian carcinoma obstruction merits admission. In this particular malignancy it does not necessarily herald end-stage disease, nor is such obstruction irreversible or even beyond chemotherapy. If the patient can be put under the care of a specialist gynaecological oncologist, so much the better.
2. A patient with gastric outlet obstruction or upper gut obstruction should usually be hospitalized. The former is diagnosed from the history of painless vomiting, after which the patient temporarily feels much more comfortable, and often wants to eat a good meal. There is minimal nausea except immediately prior to another violent vomit. These patients need gastric aspiration, possibly IV fluids, and may be candidates even at an advanced stage in their illness for a gastrojejunostomy, radiotherapy to the porta hepatis, occasionally H_2 antagonist by injection and, in the hands of a surgeon able to do the procedure speedily under ultrasound, a percutaneous jejunostomy.
3. Most patients with a lower gut obstruction should be, and can be, kept at home. They do not need 'drip and suction' but can be kept remarkably comfortable for two months or more without pain or electrolyte imbalance, provided good mouth care is given and satisfactory intake is achieved by sucking iced cubes. If they are admitted to hospital as a routine, it is almost inevitable that the junior doctor will, as he has been taught to do, have a tube down and a drip up before anyone notices that the patient is terminally ill, and these tubes will then become an unnecessary barrier between patient and family.
4. Pain is seldom very severe. The best antispasmodics are *not* pethidine (never used in modern palliative care) or the opioids, but rather hyoscine butylbromide and a prostaglandin biosynthetase inhibitor such as diclofenac. The former can be given via a syringe-driver in a dose of 20–120 milligram per day, the latter by injection or suppository.

5 Hospitals, hospices, and other help

Looking after a terminally ill person at home necessitates the members of the primary care team knowing all the local resources—hospitals, specialist clinics and services, hospices, home care services, and support agencies. One theme of this book is anticipation—planning, practising, and being proactive rather than reactive. Knowing these resources is one aspect of this exercise.

HOSPITALS

There is much to be said for a patient being able to return, when necessary, to a familiar ward of a hospital near home, possibly the unit where he was first diagnosed or where most of the definitive treatment has been given. The staff, the routine, and the surroundings are familiar, and therefore that little bit less frightening. Probably the last paragraph of each letter from the consultant has said something to the effect 'If we can help at any time, or you would like us to admit for terminal care, we should be delighted to do so'.

The sincerity of that is not in doubt. The problem, as every family doctor knows, is that that ward may not be accepting admissions when the patient needs one, or may be full, and the patient has to go to a different ward, or even a totally strange hospital, to be transferred later if fit to travel. More importantly, the doctor may have some doubts whether or not that ward is now the best place for his patient. A frenetically busy surgical ward was exhilarating and even encouraging for the patient recovering from his cancer operation but will it be able to provide what he needs now? It is not a criticism but a realistic question to ask if the brilliant surgeon who looked after the patient months or years ago is the right person to coordinate palliative care when no more surgery is possible. Is the oncology ward the appropriate place if there is not to be any more radiotherapy or chemotherapy, or the cardiology ward when no more sophisticated investigations or treatment are appropriate? The answer is, 'possibly', but the question must be asked, and asked *before* any crisis develops. It is a matter for team discussion with a unique opportunity for the community nurse to contribute from her conversations with patient and family.

As part of advanced planning of care, the team must know where would be best for each possible eventuality. Where would be best should he develop a spinal cord compression—a neurosurgery ward, an orthopaedic one, or the regional radiotherapy centre? If an AIDS patient needs sophisticated investigation and treatment for yet another infection, should he go back to an AIDS

Unit or the nearby Infectious Diseases ward? Should the patient with motor neurone disease (MND) return to the neurology ward?

We all know how every experienced family doctor gets to know the local consultants and their many qualities (and even some failings). He or she becomes adept at choosing the most suitable one for the different needs and personalities of his patients. The situation is no different for his terminally ill patients. No matter how genuine is the invitation to send a patient back to the unit, the doctor will ask himself and his colleagues who and where is best for the patient *now*.

HOSPICES

Gone are the days when hospices were where people went to die! Most are now better and more correctly described as palliative care units geared to relieving suffering and rehabilitating patients so far as is possible. Most can quote 40—70 per cent discharge rates, with hundreds of patients going in and out many times in the last year or so of life. The larger ones will be staffed by consultants in palliative medicine and with an appropriately high. nurse:patient ratio to enable them to offer high quality personalized care. On staff will be physiotherapists, occupational therapists, social workers, pastoral care workers and, freely available at short notice, lawyers and accountants able to offer their expert services.

The doctor who wants to offer the best to his patients will have familiarized himself with the local hospice and his opposite numbers there. He will know the referral and admission procedures, know their priorities for admission and, with nursing colleagues, will have visited it to see the facilities to judge if they are appropriate for some patients and possibly not for others.

A good hospice should pose no threat to general practice. It is there to support and complement good practice, but it is only as good as its staff and the standard of cooperation developed with local primary care teams.

Late referrals to a hospice are not to be recommended. They do not permit the development of good staff and patient trust and respect, and can too readily reinforce the notion of them as 'death houses' if patients are admitted within days of death. Far better for patients to be referred for hospice care when palliation is the aim rather than terminal care. Family doctors sometimes forget how comforting it can be to have a palliative medicine specialist see the patient at home, or as a hospice out-patient, and have their management endorsed by the 'expert'. They can then feel that everything which can and should be done is, in fact, being done.

SPECIALIST HOME CARE SERVICES

Not only in Britain, but in many other countries, there are now increasing numbers of such services. In Britain they may be called 'Macmillan Services' because original funding came from the Cancer Relief Macmillan Fund though they are not administered by that Fund.

Many are based on hospices or palliative care units but increasingly they are based on hospitals and, in particular, oncology units. Some are staffed entirely by nurses, each of whom is experienced not only in hospital but also community practice, with additional qualifications in oncology, palliative care, and often counselling. Other services are staffed by such nurses but have a doctor working with them, someone with considerable experience and expertise in palliative medicine, possibly even a consultant.

Each family doctor should endeavour to get to know the local team; know how, when, and why to refer to it for help; and take full advantage of their expertise. Almost universally such teams are advisory, complementing the work of primary care teams and not offering 'hands-on' care. Used properly, they do not pose any threat to good primary care teams but can bring a rich, added dimension to this work. It has to be remembered that the average family doctor only has 10—20 terminally ill patients under his care at home each year, whereas most specialist home care services will be involved with 400—500 annually, some with very many more than that.

It cannot be denied that some *do* regard them as a threat. Almost inevitably, specialist palliative care colleagues may come across a symptom which can be more adequately palliated and on many occasions, because of their training, they may identify stresses and strains not previously noted. With good working relationships and mutual respect, these can lead to the improved care of patients and relatives everyone aims to achieve.

Early referral is, once again, the best for all concerned, remembering that any home care service worthy of its good reputation will be ready to withdraw at any time if its input is no longer necessary or deemed helpful. If it is remembered that their role is to help with *palliation* rather than 'care of the dying', such services will come to be seen as less threatening to patients, less a reminder of what lies ahead. Experience shows that most patients are immensely grateful for their involvement though many relatives, probably choosing to believe the fearful diagnosis and prognosis are still not recognized by the patient, will be anxious about or resistant to their being called in—'Won't that upset him when he knows where they come from?'. Long experience suggests that these are the patients who often meet the palliative medicine consultant with, 'I've been hoping for ages you would be called in because I knew you could help!'.

DAY HOSPICES

Many British hospices operate day units, but they are less common in many other parts of the world, though steadily increasing in number. Like similar services for geriatric and psychiatric patients, they cater for those who are at home but still fit enough to be brought into a day unit on a few days each week. They are usually staffed by nurses, occupational therapists and physiotherapists, and specially selected and trained volunteers, often with back-up medical support and access to social workers, chaplains, counsellors, and others.

One almost has to see a day hospice in order to appreciate its uniquely positive atmosphere, otherwise it could sound negative and morbid if one remembers that all attending have advanced, life-threatening illness. The atmosphere is always relaxed and informal, as homely as it can possibly be. Contrary to what might be thought, its aim is not to divert patients' attention from the seriousness of their condition, but rather to focus on what can be done to improve the quality of their lives. Activities are skilfully tailored to each person's needs and abilities. Some just want to sit and watch, other to talk or be entertained, whilst most others relish developing old hobbies and skills or even taking on something quite new. One may find a man taking up carpentry or model-making, or learning how to do enamel work or pottery so that he can take home a present for his wife. Near him may be someone learning painting or cake-decorating, someone being shown how to work a computer, or another developing a stamp collection. The afternoon may be the time for entertainers, local actors or musicians, or singing by a school choir. On better days everyone may be taken out for a pub lunch or a visit to gardens, museum, or a visiting cruise ship. The casual visitor will find it difficult to realize just how ill these people are— terminally ill they may be, but all around is activity, laughter, and *living*. It has rightly been said that day hospices are not preparation for dying but reaffirm- ation of living. On the day that the author wrote this chapter, a woman told him that she had never laughed so much or enjoyed herself so much, yet she and her family all knew she only had weeks to live.

The benefits extend far beyond the patient. Caring relatives are released from their duties for a few hours to do shopping, visit the hairdresser, or just do nothing! The 'death and dying stigma' of the hospice is immediately erased and soon patient and relatives come to regard it as a positive place rather than one to be feared.

The primary care team members soon learn how to use it. They can identify those who need to be taken out of their homes which have come to feel like prison cells, patients who have become introspective and morbid, and relatives who need a well-earned break if they are to keep their loved one at home much longer. Doctors learn how to telephone the day hospice with updated informa- tion and insight into the patient's problems, or with requests that a medical colleague see the person in the day hospice and advise on palliation and support.

Those who might benefit from a few days' admission can readily be admitted and, when the time comes for final admission, there is usually no hesitation or apprehension on the part of patient or family.

PAIN RELIEF CLINIC

Such clinics are increasingly available worldwide, usually under the direction of specially trained anaesthetists supported where possible by clinical psychologists, neurologists, radiologists, and physiotherapists. Sadly, some are under-staffed and under-funded, with long waiting lists.

The days are long gone when their work consisted principally or exclusively of performing a range of sophisticated nerve blocking procedures. These form but a small part of their present-day practice, much of it being skilled diagnosis of intractable pain problems, the use of adjuvant analgesics which may be relatively unfamiliar to most doctors, and psychological techniques to assist these patients. Some clinics insist that all diagnostic work-up has been completed before they see a patient.

The problem for most family doctors looking after terminally ill patients is to know who to refer and for what indications. Some guidelines are suggested here.

1. If in any doubt about referring a patient, first have a word with the local palliative medicine specialist. If pharmacological management of the pain is possible, he will be the colleague best able to help. Similarly he is the best person, in association with physiotherapists, to advise on the use of trans-cutaneous electrical nerve stimulation (TENS), and may well be able to make appropriate equipment available on loan.
2. Consider the pain clinic for pain secondary to carcinoma of the pancreas when a coeliac plexus block may be appropriate.
3. Remember the undoubted place of percutaneous cordotomy (PCC) for patients with such unilateral pain as femoral or sciatic neuropathy or brachial plexopathy secondary to a Pancoast tumour.
4. Make early referral for the patient with cranial neuropathy such as trigeminal neuralgia where blocks can be dramatically effective.
5. The patient with bilateral pain from pelvic pathology, particularly in the lower lumbar and sacral dermatomes, may benefit from stereotactic thal-amotomy or myelotomy.
6. The patient whose pain might be expected to respond to modern pharmacological regimens but has not done so may benefit from expert psychological advice, bio-feedback, or new coping strategies, and should be referred.

COMMUNITY PHYSIOTHERAPY

Incredibly, there are still some who feel that physiotherapy has little to offer the terminally ill patient. The reason is probably they have not considered the possible benefits until the patient is too frail to benefit! As so often in palliative care, the sooner needs are reviewed and help called in, the better.

The physiotherapist can do so much for those having difficulty expectorating, or who are not aware of how to breathe correctly with their limited respiratory function. He or she can teach others how to rise from a chair, transfer from bed/chair to commode or toilet, how to walk with appropriate aids, and how to get in and out of cars. Equally important, the physiotherapist can demonstrate to relatives how to lift the patient without hurting themselves, how to mobilize people, and how to make them comfortable when in pain.

In recent years, hundreds of physiotherapists have learned the new technique for the management and reduction of lymphoedema, doing away with such equipment as Flowtron or Jobst inflated compression sleeves. The sooner such patients are referred, the better. The results can be remarkable. Most palliative care units have specialist physiotherapists skilled in this technique or can advise where to send such a patient.

'COMPLEMENTARY' THERAPIES

Confusion inevitably exists about what constitutes 'complementary' and 'alternative' therapies. The author's views are his own and not likely to meet with universal agreement!

1. Acupuncture has a real place in palliative care. It may be recommended by a palliative medicine consultant or a pain specialist and its benefits are well proven for a few conditions. Like anything else in medicine, it is not a panacea.
2. Hynotherapy is similar in its place. Performed by a medical hypnotherapist, and not a theatrical showman, hypnosis can relax a patient (who may sometimes be able to learn autohypnosis, often using an audio tape) and can sometimes be helpful as a means of exploring deep, unexpressed fears and phobias.
3. Aromatherapy is increasingly learned and practised by many in palliative care who are convinced of its therapeutic benefits. The author, however, has yet to be convinced and looks forward to seeing the results of controlled studies which clearly demonstrate that benefit is related to the specific aroma and not the understandable comfort of a caring, gentle person devoting so much time to the patient as an aromatherapist always does. Even if scientific tests fail to substantiate the claims, no one can deny the benefits of time being devoted to these patients and addressing their previously unmet needs.

What should be the family doctor's response to someone who wants to go outside traditional medical care for help, whatever form it takes? Surely the answer must be to advise on any benefits and any dangers and to let them go if they wish. In addition, one must always remind them that no one blames them, and that they can return unashamed and unembarrassed at any time, but that the doctor would like to be kept informed of where they are going and what they are taking.

COOPERATING WITH COLLEAGUES

The experienced family doctor does not need to be reminded that one of his difficult and delicate tasks is referring to other colleagues, whether they are hospital or hospice colleagues, or many of the others described in this chapter. In a sense he is the professional guardian and advocate of his patient, whom he has probably known for a long time and many of whose relatives will continue under his care for years to come.

The reasons for, and the timing of, referrals are crucial. Too late a referral runs the risk of some problems not being adequately handled, whilst too early a referral might be misinterpreted by patient and family as the doctor's inability or inexperience or, worse still, disinterest in continuing to care for the patient at home. Sometimes help is needed as much for the family as for the patient, but they may not wish to hear this. Referral to the wrong colleague or agency can waste precious time and upset all concerned.

The answer lies in the skilled planning and coordination of palliative care. Only when the whole complex picture is examined by the doctor, partners, nurses, and ancillary staff is it possible to define the issues, set priorities, allocate responsibilities, and decide when additional help could benefit all concerned. Rarely are the wrong decisions made after such thorough team assessments and reviews. It is when the reactive doctor comes across a problem which could have been anticipated and dealt with earlier, that inappropriate referrals tend to be made.

Some might say that it is easier said than done, but the ideal is for the doctor to telephone his opposite number in hospital, hospice, or clinic and discuss the issues with him. It then becomes easier to decide where is best, who can offer the appropriate care, and how it should be explained, with the family doctor remaining 'in control' at all times and giving the necessary confidence to patient, family, and colleagues in the primary care team.

6 Aids, appliances, and equipment

Caring for a terminally ill person at home may call for extra aids, appliances, and equipment to be made available, and members of the primary health care team must know of them, their indications, and availability. Research has shown that many relatives are not told of them, or only informed late in the illness when they could have made all the difference if provided earlier. An appraisal of such needs should form part of the routine team review of care being offered for each patient.

It must also be stressed, for the sake of relatives and the professionals themselves, that the dying rarely if ever need 'special' equipment different from that needed by any other ill patients under care at home, contrary to what some relatives may suspect.

In this chapter, different pieces of equipment are described but few details given about where they may be borrowed or bought because this inevitably varies from country to country, and district to district.

SPECIAL MATTRESSES

The prevention of pressure sores in the terminally ill is difficult, the cure of them almost impossible. (Because so much of the final year is spent at home, 80 per cent of bedsores start there.) Too often attention is first given to this problem when the skin has already broken and the patient is suffering pain which is more persistent and upsetting than many cancer pains and almost resistant to analgesics.

No one piece of equipment meets all needs and nothing can replace the regular and skilled attention of a community nurse or relatives taught the principles of skin care. When it is recognized that a patient may have to sit or lie for prolonged periods—no matter how long the life expectancy is thought to be or what the underlying pathology is—the community nurse should become involved in the care, and not merely when sores are established.

Ripple or bubble mattresses are very popular, the former having transverse ridges which inflate and deflate in turn to prevent the patient's weight being directed for long on any one area. The bubble mattress is possibly superior with its surface of palm-sized pockets of air. The model preferred by most palliative care nursing specialists, though usually more expensive, is the Spenco mattress or chair cushion, easy to wash and exceedingly comfortable for patients. An alternative for chairs and wheelchairs is the Roho, ugly and uncomfortable in appearance but very acceptable when it is correctly inflated for the individual patient.

SHEEPSKIN COVERS

Usually made of synthetic fibre rather than natural sheepskin, these come in different sizes for chairs and beds, the latter either large enough for the whole bed or sufficient for the area of most pressure. They are easily washed but inevitably lose some of their 'fluffiness' in time. Some patients, particularly those perspiring with advanced cancer, find them too hot. Unless instructed in their use, some relatives may put them under the drawsheet rather than immediately under the patient.

TRIANGULAR (DELTA) PILLOWS

These clumsy-looking pillows, firmly filled to offer maximum support, are a boon to the dyspnoeic patient with chronic obstructive pulmonary disease who otherwise slips down on ordinary pillows, or possibly cannot afford all the extra pillows needed to be kept comfortably propped up in bed. They are less commonly needed for patients with malignant chest conditions and may be uncomfortable for the patient with skin secondaries from a squamous cell bronchogenic carcinoma or mesothelioma.

TABLE FAN

Whilst it is certainly true that oxygen is not often needed, and only then for the patient with clinical anoxia, the psychological effect of a table fan blowing cool air around the dyspnoeic patient cannot be denied. It has the added advantage of being easy to move to whichever chair or room the patient is in and is always under his or her own control.

DEODORIZERS

The eradication or reduction of unpleasant odours is not always easy but is of considerable importance for many patients and their relatives at home. Few carers will admit that the smell emanating from a loved one is so bad they want him or her removed to hospital, but many will later admit they found it upsetting or even nauseatingly offensive.

The malodour from an ileostomy or colostomy can be reduced by employing the special charcoal inserts advised by the ostomy manufacturers. That of fungating tumours can be much reduced with topical metronidazole gel or, if this is not available or is too expensive as in some countries, metronidazole pessaries can be flaked and crushed and mixed with a lubricant jelly such as KY Jelly. On top of all dressings, held in place by the external bandage, can be placed an activated charcoal pad changed daily (Actasorb or Denidor).

Portable electric charcoal deodorizers can be obtained on loan or purchase for the sick room or an ultraviolet deodorizer (as used in some food shops) fitted to a wall or cupboard.

Contrary to what might be thought, the type of household aerosol air fresheners, so generally available, are not to be recommended. Their scent soon becomes nauseating and may forever after be associated by the relatives with the suffering and death of their loved one.

TOILET APPLIANCES

The time to provide a commode is when the patient begins to feel that the toilet is much further away than it used to be, not when he needs assistance to get there or has fallen on one of his attempts to do so. Dying should not become an endurance test or obstacle race!

The choice of commode is important. Does it need a backrest or arms (fixed or removable)? Should it be a chemical commode (when there are not relatives able or willing to empty it)? Which member of the care team will instruct the relatives on its cleaning and disinfecting? Who will show them how the patient can be transferred from bed or chair to the commode? Have they been reassured that the urine or faeces do not contain disease, even cancer, because experience suggests many relatives do harbour this fear of cancer transmission?

The patients still able to use the household toilet may need a special fitting to elevate it for easier use, or special padding, or the provision of handrails to facilitate easier and safer getting on and off it. In the United Kingdom such modifications are arranged through the community occupational therapy services.

BATH AIDS

Many patients prefer to struggle on, bathing themselves as long as possible before finally accepting the offer of a community nurse to assist them, yet we are all aware of the relative ease of getting into a bath and the considerable effort needed to get out of one. They can be helped by the provision of special bath seats, handrails fixed between taps to grip as they get up, and non-slip mats. Other useful aids are hair-rinse showers fixed to the taps and a long-handled back-scrubber to help them feel independent.

In many countries showers are more popular than baths but they, too, can be dangerous without support rails and non-slip mats to stand on, and unless care is taken to ensure that temperature control is simple and safe, particularly for hands crippled with rheumatism.

The experienced family doctor knows that having the community nurse help with bathing can often be the best way to introduce her to the patient, getting frailer yet proudly holding on to independence in other areas.

WHEELCHAIRS

To order a wheelchair one needs to know the patient's height, length of thigh and breadth of hips, with an estimate of the patient's weight. The supplier must also be told whether it is to be self-propelling (rarely appropriate for the patients we are discussing) or to be collapsible to fit into a car boot. Other refinements to be considered are whether there needs to be a high back, whether it should be able to be tilted, whether leg extensions are needed because of knee stiffness or arthrodesis, and whether arms, foot rests, and even back need to be removable.

Once again, the care team must decide who is to instruct patients and relatives in its use. The necessary skills are rarely inborn!

NYLON LADDER

This is a simple but valuable device, wooden spars linked like a ladder by nylon ropes which can easily be tied to the bedframe so that the patient can pull himself up in bed without having to trouble a relative. Provided the patient has reasonable arm and shoulder girdle muscle, it is much easier and safer to use than a 'monkey-pole' hanging over the bed.

COMMUNICATION AIDS

These can make all the difference to patients with communication difficulties whether secondary to CVAs, cerebral metastases, MND, or other pathology. The simplest, provided the patient can point to his need, is a card on which are drawn such items as a glass of water, a urinal, a toilet, a book etc.

More sophisticated, much more expensive, but invaluable, are electronic aids of various kinds. Some are like miniature typewriters which display the words typed (and may then vocalize them via an electronic voice) or print them out like a teleprinter. Some, like the Possum, obtainable via rehabilitation or neurology services, can be operated by fingers, tongue, lips or even breath (see Figure 6.1).

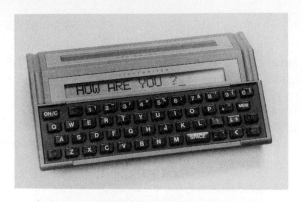

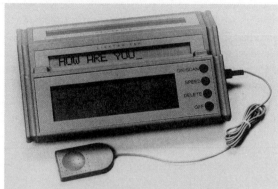

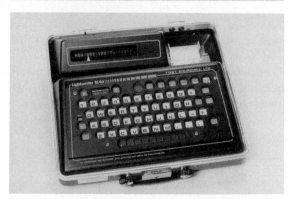

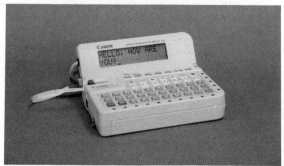

Fig. 6.1 Communication aids: Lightwriter SL8, Lightwriter SL30, Lightwriter SL4A, Canon Communicator.

It is imperative to assess the patient's needs as early in the condition as possible, not when they are exhausted, frightened, and dejected by their disability, and to involve the specialist help of a speech therapist for expert advice. Only such an authority can adequately assess and advise on appropriate communication aids.

LIQUIDIZER

We all know how important it is for patients with Celestin or Atkinson tubes to have attractively-served liquidized food, but many others can benefit—those with oesophageal strictures, those with neuromuscular dysfunctions, others too tired to enjoy normal meals, and the very elderly. The important thing to remember is that 'normal' food can look appallingly unattractive when meat, vegetables, and gravy are all liquidized together and presented in one dish. Using separate little dishes, each with a touch of colour (mint, parsley, red pepper, sauce, or ketchup) can make all the difference.

VACUUM FLASKS

Many ill patients can safely be left at home for an hour or two while a relative goes out to work or shop, provided food and drinks are left within easy reach and the patient is fit enough to handle them. The secret is to have small flasks light enough to hold and open, for hot and cold drinks, and others with wide tops for soup, ice cream or sorbet, or other nourishing snacks, with a supply of plastic spoons rather than metal knives and forks.

FIRE-RESISTANT APRONS

The patient who insists on smoking, yet is scarcely able to hold his cigarette or pipe, or keeps falling asleep whilst smoking, can be a danger to himself and the whole household. Special fire-resistant aprons can be purchased and tied onto the patient or bed by tapes, or simply draped across his knees. In the United Kingdom they are obtainable from Tutor Safety Products, Sturminster Newton, Dorset DT10 1BZ.

RADIO, TV, AND TAPES

We all know the pleasure patients get from TV, radio, and listening to tapes and CDs. How can they enjoy them without disturbing others in the home and, equally important, how can they be protected from the noise of the family TV or radio in the adjoining room? So many appliances are now available but, for some reason, many relatives seem to lack imagination and common sense in this matter.

For example, it is useful if the patient's TV can have a remote control to save having to call family to change channels, and even more useful if either the patient's TV or another one in the house can be adapted so that sound is only heard via lightweight earphones.

There are now relatively cheap tape and cassette players with comfortable ear/headphones which can enable the patient to enjoy favourite music, plays, and readings, without disturbing or being disturbed by others. Another useful device is a small earpiece which can be placed under the pillows so that relaxing music can be heard only by the patient, lying comfortably on their pillows in bed.

If a music therapist is available, they can be of inestimable value, advising on suitable music, making tapes of favourite tunes, all to suit mood and need.

SPECIAL ARMCHAIRS

The frailer the patient, the more difficulty they will experience in rising from a chair, no matter how comfortable it is. No longer being able to get up unaided from the favourite chair is not an indication for permanent bedrest, but for the timely provision of a higher chair, preferably with a high back and padded arms. Even better is an electric model which can be controlled by the patient to alter height, angle, etc.

Even an ordinary chair can be made more suitable by the provision of a spring-seat fitting which pushes the person up when they lean forward and upwards, saving strain on the pelvic girdle. Many good furniture manufacturers can advise on such models. The best professional advice can be obtained through community occupational services.

LAP-TOP TRAYS

These trays, usually with a heat-resistant, non-slip surface, rest easily on a person's knees, whether in chair or bed, by moulding the bag of plastic balls in the attached cushion. They are relatively cheap, make it possible for the patient to have food and drink without spilling, and can be purchased in many shops or through the occupational therapy services.

7 Spiritual issues

Often 'spirituality' is confused with 'religion' and 'faith'. They are not synonymous. Spirituality means 'the search for existential meaning', a somewhat grand way to describe an experience common to us all at different times of life. Unless we recognize spiritual issues and separate them from religious ones, we shall fail to help some patients, arguing that a person's religion is a very personal and intimate matter, not an area into which a doctor should intrude and certainly not invade by proselytizing.

Man's search for existential meaning describes his constantly asking, 'Why?'. Why does Man suffer? What is the meaning of life? Why do some suffer more in life than others? Do our lives, and how we live them, matter? Is there a God? Does He care, does He even know what goes on, and does He answer prayer? Is there life after death and, if so, what will it be like? The list is endless. Is there anyone who has not asked these questions?

The answer is probably that many do not ask such questions when life is going well, when they are happy and healthy. They *do* ask them when they are ill, their lives are under threat and possibly likely to come to a premature end, with ambitions unfulfilled, relationships strained, differences not resolved, and hopes dashed. In fact, more than 75 per cent of dying people speak of them, given the opportunity. Do we give *our* patients this opportunity?

It is natural to ask these questions when bodily health is failing, energy lessening, and every facet of life changing almost daily. The young man soon to leave wife and children and all he had dreamt of is bound to ask 'Why?'. The frail, elderly person, who has always relished helping others and now is totally dependent on others for every activity of daily living, inevitably asks why they go on living a life they now find a burden, apparently of no use to anyone. The person with a lifelong faith asks why their God lets them suffer and wonders if He knows how they feel or if He is punishing them.

As the end of life approaches, many people discover things about themselves they never knew before. They gain insights into their personality and character which may disturb them. They find their faith or philosophy has been immature or inadequate, their courage or their decisiveness nonexistent. The man who prided himself on his macho image comes to appreciate how dependent he has always been on a wife whom he had often regarded as helpless and indecisive, a wife whom he could have loved and respected more.

It might be thought, or indeed expected, that those with a faith would find the final months of life less fearful or upsetting than those without such a faith. This is not always so. Some have never thought about death and its implications.

Others have had what one can only describe as too simplistic or immature a faith, or perhaps one which has seldom been tested. Yet others find it difficult to understand God's ways or even to articulate prayers. It is, for example, a common experience for a terminally ill person to say the Lord's Prayer but studiously leave unsaid the words 'Thy will be done'. Some find it difficult to reconcile God's concern for them and their loved ones and His taking them away through death.

GUIDELINES FOR ASSISTING WITH SPIRITUAL PROBLEMS

1. The family doctor, particularly if he works in a village, small town or circumscribed area, is often well placed to know and to speak to local clergy. He may even know if his patient is a Church member. After broaching the subject with the patient, he can usefully contact the clergyman and invite him to share in the patient's care. This means much more than intimating how ill the person is. It is a recognition that both have much to offer, much to share, for that patient's good—the doctor and the clergyman. It implies something which is often missing, namely mutual respect for each other's role, respect for confidentiality, and compassionate concern. Primary care teams can easily overlook the fact that clergy often have deep knowledge and understanding of patients and their families built up over years. They have ministered to them 'in sickness and in health', seen their strengths as well as their weaknesses, and can often help not only the patient but also the health professionals with their insight. It is salutary to remember that in the last 20 years newly ordained clergy have had much more training on grief, bereavement, stress, and coping mechanisms than most medical students and nurses have!

2. Do not fall into the trap of trying to answer spiritual and philosophical questions of the patient. When someone asks why God does something, or what God is thinking about, much as he might like to know the answer he does not really think his highly respected and intelligent family doctor will know the mind of God!

3. Do not offer trite platitudes! No matter how well-intentioned, whatever is said is not likely to be helpful. What may sound to the doctor and nurse like a clever response will not impress the patient who is far more likely to be comforted by knowing that no one else has an answer, yet everyone keeps asking the same profound questions. It is very similar to bereavement counselling. The best counsellors are those who can listen without feeling they must speak. Even the most well-meant comment or response is likely to be misunderstood and even hurtful. Though not intended to be trite, it can so easily sound it.

4. You should not proselytize but, at the same time, if the doctor or nurse has a faith it can help others to know this, and even to learn how such a faith can still be supportive without providing all the answers. Perhaps we forget that our modern society seems to expect answers to every question, and solutions to every problem. Experience shows that many patients are actually helped by hearing that their doctor does not know everything or that, very real as his faith is to him, he too occasionally asks the same questions and has the same problems. 'I'm like you—I don't know why this happens, I wish I did—but I'm still sure there is a God who cares even though I can't understand Him.'

5. Be sensitive to the person who always found comfort in prayer and now finds it difficult to know what to say and even why to pray. So many regard prayer as a list of requests to God rather than a two-way conversation with Him. We can reassure them that they are not unusual (most very ill people experience this) and it does not betoken a loss of faith or anything of which to be ashamed. It is, however, something to mention to the clergyman or pastoral care worker if the patient consents.

6. Respect customs and practices which mean much to the patient but perhaps nothing to the carers. There may be no medical explanation for benefit from anointing with oil or taking holy water or the receiving of the Sacraments, but who are we to dismiss anything which bring comfort and meaning to a dying patient. Even more is this the case when looking after someone of a different faith or from a different cultural background.

7. Praying, or looking, for a cure does not imply that the patient has not understood or accepted the diagnosis. This should not lead the doctor or nurse to give more explicit explanations because the patient is in a stage of 'denial'.

8. Remember the bewilderment of relatives when they find their loved one asking spiritual questions after a lifetime without any expression of faith or interest in such profound issues. They may ask if it is a feature of the illness, if he is mentally disturbed, or even if it is a side-effect of his drugs. They will probably find it even more trying because their own faith may be wilting (hopefully temporarily) during this crisis.

How then, recognizing that in each of us there is a spiritual dimension, can the doctor or nurse help the patient whether or not these issues are ever articulated?

1. We can train ourselves to recognize spiritual problems in the same way every family doctor or community nurse aims to recognize pain or fear without the patient mentioning them. If not articulated they may present as defeatism, 'face to the wall', depression without most of the usual clinical features of a depressive state (particularly 'hopelessness'), surprising tension between a previously well-balanced couple, physical symptoms not responding as

expected, fears or tension the patient cannot explain . . . There are, as yet, no well-defined syndromes. We must simply be aware of this dimension of life and be as ready to become involved as we would with pain, anxiety, or social issues.

2. We can positively broach the subject with the patient, not by way of direct interrogation as in history-taking, but almost as an aside. 'Do you ever find yourself asking why this is happening—why me?' 'I suppose you do a lot of thinking now that you have to sit so much?' 'I wouldn't be surprised if, even with that faith I know you have, you find it being taxed at this time?' 'You may have no pain now and be looking a bit better, but I suppose there are other problems you wish were as easy to solve?'

3. We can sit and share our humanity with the patient! How readily we forget that whilst we see ourselves as highly qualified professionals, our patients would prefer to see us as friends, and good friends can make us feel better just by five minutes sitting quietly together. Even the busy family doctor can take five minutes off his coffee break to sit with a dying friend. An anecdote beloved by the author is of an old, very quietly religious lady near the end of life. When asked how the author could help her, she suggested he buy a platform ticket—a reminder of the days when, with such a ticket, one could wait on the railway platform to see a friend off on their journey. With gentle humour she told what it felt like to have a one-way ticket, to be going some-where—like a travel brochure, it sounded attractive, but she had not met anyone who had been there, and how typical of British Rail for her train to be late! Days and days passed without her wishing to trouble the author until at last she called him over. 'The train's coming and, you know, I am both excited and apprehensive but quite lonely. Please stay with me and see me off.' A few minutes later she said, 'You can't come any further with me, I'll be alright' and died.

4. We can help our patients to see their contribution to life, because so many people die wondering if the world will miss them, if they have achieved or contributed anything. Ask them to tell you of their family, of their Army service, of the biggest decisions or crises in life—it soon becomes obvious that their life has not been without worth and they need to be shown that. Some people benefit from being invited to record or write their memoirs. Others need to make a tape for the family they are leaving behind. All need to know that they have been useful and are still needed right to the end. We all want to feel we shall be missed.

5. We should never forget to thank our patients for what they are doing, and have done, to make us more caring doctors and nurses. Each patient, in one way or another, increases our knowledge and understanding, but they will never even suspect that unless we tell them.

Dying need not be a time of loss and defeat. It can be a time for remembering, a time for forgiving, and even a time for final growth. Our task as doctors and nurses is to help make this possible. We can be highly skilled 'symptomato-logists' who ease pain but remain aloof and all-knowing, or we can be their friends, the companions who join them for part of a final journey of discovery, companions on the loneliest journey of life.

8 Ethical issues

There are no ethical medical or nursing issues peculiar to palliative care. Many, however, come into sharper focus at this time in a patient's care. There are excellent books and papers written on medical ethics in general and on the ethical issues of palliative care in particular. This chapter will focus exclusively on the issues as encountered by primary care teams providing domiciliary palliative care.

CONFIDENTIALITY

A professional involved in the care of a patient, whether terminally ill or not, has a duty and a responsibility not to divulge any information about that patient to any third party without the explicit consent of the patient. By tradition and universal acceptance, it is regarded as permissible to pass on to fellow professionals sharing in his or her care relevant information which might assist them.

This sound straightforward, but every doctor and nurse knows how frequently they are expected to break this rule and, incidentally, how easy it is to do so. Relatives and other carers pressurize them for what, to them, sound good compassionate reasons. They want to shield or protect the patient yet themselves be as fully informed as possible to help in their caring and planning for the future.

The problem rarely starts when palliative care commences. Most people ask that the diagnosis be withheld from the patient when it is first made and then continue to 'protect' him as they see fit. Even when, as most studies have continued to demonstrate, the patient knew all along both the diagnosis and prognosis, these relatives refuse to believe this and go to great lengths to keep the truth from them. Often this becomes a charade, both parties convincing themselves that the other does not know. Usually the patient does not declare how much he knows, even to his doctor. The relatives expect to be told everything whilst denying the patient his or her basic right to information about their life, their illness, and its care, and ultimately about their dying.

The professionals cannot, must not, allow themselves to be drawn into this conspiracy of silence. In the most courteous yet firm manner they must explain how the patient has a right to all information he or she wants, and further explain the undoubted benefits of keeping trust with him — equally, the problems which may arise from deception and half-truths. The family doctor, with his accepted authority in the home, must be able to keep the patient informed and to dissuade the family from asking for details not yet given to the patient. The community nurse may not fare so well. She is perceived as more approachable and more understanding of their position. Going downstairs after attending to her patient, she is often invited into the family circle and asked for details of the illness, the prognosis, explanations of what doctor has said, her opinion about alternative regimens—some of which the patient is not privy to or not given permission to discuss.

It cannot be stressed strongly enough that, once the professionals break the rules of confidentiality and open honest communication in palliative care, the patient no longer has any good reason to trust those into whose hands he has put his life for what time is left. The many fears of the dying can only be addressed in an atmosphere of trust based on truth and mutual respect. Break that trust and a Pandora's box of troubles and fears is opened, never again to be adequately controlled.

The need for regular, frequent meetings of the doctors and nurses involved in the care cannot be exaggerated. Each must know what the other has said, what relatives have asked and been told, and each must trust and respect the judgement and actions of fellow professionals working in the team.

NUTRITION AND REHYDRATION

Dietary issues are the subject of Chapter 3. Here we are considering how to respond to demands for such procedures as total parenteral nutrition (TPN) and intravenous rehydration. These demands are made by relatives (often at odds with other members of the family) who see these not as means of bringing about comfort in the final weeks but as life-sustaining measures—desperate, but in their minds, totally justifiable means of holding onto their loved one as long as possible. The assumption, of course, is that the patient's steady decline is not due to the underlying disease process but to starvation, dehydration, or medical inactivity.

There is nothing wrong with TPN or IV fluid replacement. Both have a place in medical care. The issue here is to decide when they are appropriate and when not, and how to explain this to all concerned so that they see such a decision as being based on sound clinical judgement, not professional disinterest or defeatism. The difficulty in explaining a decision not to embark on either measure is complicated when the patient has clearly benefitted in the past from TPN or infusions. On those occasions, he may have been seen by the family as dying, then apparently 'brought back to life' by these measures. Why not do it again now?

The doctor (hopefully with his or her nurse colleague) must first deliberate carefully whether either measure might help the patient. If so, they should discuss it with a specialist colleague before saying anything to the patient and family. If it is thought inappropriate they must explain their reasoning to all concerned and not hesitate to invoke the help of a specialist who knows the patient (for example, an oncologist or palliative medicine specialist), inviting them to add weight to their advice. It often requires the family doctor's long-standing, deep knowledge of the patient and family, coupled with the specialist's experience and authority, to persuade some members of the family that TPN, dietary supplements, and/or rehydration will not add weeks, far less months or years, to the patient's life. More than that, they may further burden the patient with equipment, will almost certainly entail hospitalization, and can form a physical barrier between patient and carers.

One final cautionary note: this is one area of care where, inadvertently or carelessly, family doctors and community nurses can easily find themselves giving conflicting advice. It only needs the careless throwaway comment, 'Perhaps he's restless because he's dehydrated' or 'I wonder if he needs a blood transfusion' for the family to become confused and imagine that there is no consensus opinion amongst the carers. Equally, it is irresponsible for a patient to be sent to hospital with an implied promise that a drip will be set up or something be given 'to restore his appetite' when this was never the intention of the family doctor, who was actually admitting the patient to hospital or hospice for more nursing care. It is as unkind and irresponsible as sending a patient into a hospital or hospice to die, but telling the relatives that it is for 'convalescence' or 'respite', and 'He'll soon be home again'. This happens!

EUTHANASIA

Here we are not speaking of the 'gentle death' which is the true meaning of euthanasia, and surely everyone's goal. We are referring to the deliberate taking of a person's life with the intention of ending their suffering. As we all know, such an act is illegal in every country of the Western world, whether or not the patient has ever expressed a wish for it in time gone by, whether or not they were then and are now of sound mind. The act, no matter how well intentioned, amounts to murder in legal terms. It might be thought that this issue would not be raised when a patient is in the terminal phase of an illness, but this is far from true.

Every doctor will, at some time or other in his professional life, be taken aside by a relative and asked to bring the suffering to an end. Often there will be a substantial financial incentive offered, or moral pressure applied with such comments as 'You would never let your dog suffer like this', or 'You should see how much he is suffering when you are not here'. Always there is the assurance that no one need ever learn that the act had been performed.

There can only be one response: a firm, polite refusal. At the same time, the doctor must pledge himself or herself to do everything possible to relieve all suffering and so support and help the relatives and friends that they will not assuage their undoubted sorrow and pain by asking someone to commit murder on their behalf. It is worth remembering the adage that 'A plea for euthanasia is a plea for better care'. Nearly always it is found that more *can* be done to ease pain and restlessness, to aid sleep, or reduce fear. The good doctor will never be too proud to consult partners or hospital/hospice colleagues for advice.

It should be remembered that research has consistently and conclusively shown that many relatives perceive that the dying patient is suffering more pain and anxiety than is actually the case. The reasons are obvious and easy to understand. It must also be remembered that the key word in this ethical dilemma, like so many others, is *intent*. A tranquillizer can be given sufficient to sedate the patient and leave him heavily sedated and at peace, provided the *intention* was to do just that, and not in fact to terminate his life or expedite his death.

This reminds us of the vexed question of double effect so beloved of ethicists. It is sometimes argued that doctors, claiming to use the therapeutic effect of a drug, are actually taking advantage of another action which is toxic or lethal rather than therapeutic. The example most commonly given is the opioids. It is said that doctors sometimes prescribe them as analgesics, but in fact are aiming to depress respiration so that the patient will die. Some argue that even if the *intent* is not to shorten life, the fact is that they are doing so. Another group of drugs similarly implicated are the benzodiazepines. Anyone with knowledge of pharmacology will know that depression of respiration does not occur with opioids correctly prescribed for chronic pain. The same cannot be said for high-dose benzodiazepines, but here we return to this issue of *intent*. In law, if the doctor can swear that the drugs were prescribed for their sedative, tranquil-lizing, muscle-relaxing properties and not with the implied aim of depressing respiration, he is acting ethically and within the law.

Having said that, the doctor will encounter relatives who either ask that the dose be increased to shorten the end-stage of a patient's life or suspect the doctor of employing the drug for that purpose. The answer is for the doctor to keep his immediate colleagues fully informed of his therapeutic intentions, and to keep the relatives equally informed of the reasons for every single prescription and change in medication. As in so much of palliative care, problems, mis-understandings, and suspicions usually follow poor communication rather than openness and honesty.

COMMUNICATION

In palliative care, as in all medical and nursing practice, good communication is essential. More problems and difficulties arise from poor communication than from anything else.

One of the most common complaints of relatives caring for a dying loved one is that they are not kept informed. As is stated in other sections of this book, they may know the diagnosis and eventual fatal outcome but may not have been kept up-to-date with the results of investigations, the rationale for treatments, and the frequently changing priorities and prognoses. Examples abound. They know that he had radiotherapy, but not why. They presume that it was to cure, or attempt to cure, the cancer because no one explained in a way they could understand that it was to control haemoptysis or pain, or reduce tumour bulk in an obstructed bronchus, or for mediastinal adenopathy. Chemotherapy is equally, if not more, bewildering — is it to cure the malignancy or to give a longer survival? Even more basic is this need to understand the operation and what the surgeon did. Was it to remove the tumour or to palliate? When the surgeon said he 'took it all away', did he mean exactly that and, if so, why are we now, a year or two later, caring for a loved one said to be dying of widespread cancer? What did he mean when he said he 'took most of it away'? If not all, how much did he leave, and why? When, after the operation, he said the prognosis was 'anything between two weeks and two years', what did he mean? When the family doctor now talks of 'keeping him comfortable', what does he mean, and why is he now talking of asking the surgeon for more advice?

These are not hypothetical questions, nor are the examples far-fetched, as any family doctor can attest. He spends much of his life trying to interpret such explanations so that the patients and relatives will better understand, and usually he feels that he has succeeded. It is only later that he learns that his nursing colleagues have had to interpret or translate what he said, and he comes to realize that even his communication skills are not as good as he had thought.

One thing is certain. It is nearly impossible for all the professionals sharing in the care to speak with one voice so that the patient and all the relatives hear the same thing and understand it. It reminds us how important it is, in all correspondence between family doctors and hospital colleagues, to ask questions about the patient's knowledge of the condition, understanding of what has been said, the exact phrases used in describing serious illnesses, and ask how best we can help fellow professionals in this shared care and issue of communication.

ADVANCED DIRECTIVES

Particularly in North America, there is much debate about the possible benefits of legalizing so-called Advanced Directives, popularly known as 'Living Wills'. They are the witnessed and recorded wishes of a person, made at a time of health and presumed sound mind, instructing that no *extraordinary* measures be used to resuscitate them or keep them alive should they ever become so ill and frail as to lose any quality of life and become a burden on loved ones and society. Frankly, they are intended to prevent what many would describe as 'medical meddling'. The person does not wish to be kept alive artificially or to be brought back from the brink of death only to remain more dependent on others than they would wish. They have seen or heard of people maintained on life-support systems and do not want this for themselves, nor do they want the inevitable strain and stress for their loved ones.

One can well understand their fears. What is sad is that anyone should feel it necessary to go to such lengths to make their wishes known; sad to feel that doctors have so often acted without due thought to a patient's quality of life or previously expressed wishes. Have we not all at one time or another been guilty of this?

Dealing with a terminally ill person at home, this is not as difficult an issue as it might appear. The good family doctor will know his patient well and may have talked through this issue in times past. He or she can easily reassure the patient and family that there will be no 'meddling', no 'officious striving' as the patient feared. Nothing will be done to 'maintain life at all cost' but everything will certainly be done to ease suffering and respect dignity. Not only must the doctor and nurse *say* this—they must demonstrate it!

So far so good—while the patient is at home! Will the hospital doctors be in harmony with these principles if he has to be admitted for some reason? Will the family find their loved one on intravenous antibiotics or being prepared for surgery when they next visit him? Will the new and eager oncologist who has not seen him before start a new chemotherapy regimen or offer to include him in his new drug trial?

The duty of the family doctor is to ensure that the patient's wishes are made clear to all concerned by whatever means are available: letter, telephone call or, even better, a face-to-face meeting with hospital colleagues. This is particularly necessary if a patient has to be admitted to a unit where he is not known.

There will be other occasions when 'further treatment' is justified and indeed to be encouraged by the primary care team because it will improve the quality of remaining life if not extend it. This can be equally difficult to explain. Some illustrations may help. Who would wish to withhold appropriate treatment of hypercalcaemia from a patient reasonably well until days before its onset? Who would not recommend a colostomy for a patient with relatively advanced colonic carcinoma if it saved them the pain, faecal vomiting, and misery of obstruction? If there was a good chance of removing all pain with a percutaneous cordotomy, would it be right not to recommend it instead of persevering with drugs less appropriate, less effective, and more upsetting? These, and many more examples all doctors could give, are potent reminders of how flexible one must be in palliative care and how skilled, honest, and informed must be our communications with patients, families, and fellow professionals.

9 The final days

No matter how difficult, indeed impossible, it may be to give a prognosis months or even weeks before the end, it should not be difficult to recognize when the patient has only a matter of days to live. This is important because many details of the care must then be altered and a well-planned course of action followed.

Sadly, there is much evidence that this point in a patient's life is not always recognized, or indeed even looked for. The result may be a breakdown in care and an unnecessary loss of quality of life. More rarely the diagnosis of dying is made prematurely and the results are equally distressing for all concerned.

DIAGNOSING THE END PHASE

Much depends on clinical acumen at this stage. No objective test can replace it. One notices the extreme lethargy, the disinterest not only in food but in fluids, the impaired mental clarity even without frank confusion, and a remarkable serenity even in patients so recently anxious or agitated. Changes are noticed even within a day, whereas before they were observed over weeks.

The body temperature falls even when there is a slight infection, respiration becomes shallower, and Cheyne–Stokes respiration may be observed during the day rather than only at night as previously. Blood pressure falls, colour fades, and the extremities are colder. Diuretics produce less diuresis, anxiolytics and hypnotics produce a more profound effect because of reduced renal elimination, pain is less and often never reported if analgesia is satisfactory. For reasons which are not clear, oedema which may have been a major problem for some considerable time suddenly disappears.

By this stage there are no indications for investigations if everything points to the patient having only days to live. The only possible reason for doing any would be if there was any doubt about this. For example, a very rapid decline in a patient until days before reasonably well with a squamous cell bronchogenic carcinoma would suggest the possibility of hypercalcaemia, the reversal of which could give him many more weeks of good life. The sudden onset of weakness and confusion would raise the possibility of SIADH (secretion of inappropriate antidiuretic hormone), where again a treatment might be justified. Sudden weakness and collapse, with hypotension, might be hypoadrenalism (Addison's) secondary to a metastasis, adrenal haemorrhage, or failure to take appropriate doses of replacement hydrocortisone, and would respond to treatment. However, rewarding as these conditions are to diagnose and treat, they are very uncommon. They should not encourage the doctor to continue blood tests when all his energies could now be directed to reviewing the care plan with nursing colleagues.

Three things must now be done:

- review medication
- review the nursing care
- review the care of the relatives.

Review medication

Continue only the essential drugs and discontinue all others, no matter how long the patient has been on them. Essential drugs will include analgesics, anticonvulsants, and tranquillizers. It must never be forgotten that pain can be experienced even at this stage and even by a patient in stupor or coma. Such patients can still have fits and many will need tranquillizers. Nonessential drugs will include iron, vitamins, cardiac drugs, hypoglycaemic and anti-hypertensive agents, diuretics and potassium supplements, longterm antibiotics, antidepressants, and H_2 antagonists.

Review the route of administration. The oral route may only be feasible intermittently, and there is no guarantee of absorption from the gut. The rectal route may appeal as being relatively noninvasive, but its appropriateness will depend on bowel function, faecal impaction, the presence of blood and mucus, of course the patient's attitude to frequent insertion of suppositories, and whether or not it seems right to keep disturbing the patient to insert them.

Many doctors continue too long employing the oral route, supplementing it with intermittent injections. They forget that injected opioid agonists such as morphine and diamorphine need to be given every 4 hours or that IM diazepam takes so long to be effective. Rarely are general practitioners and community nurses able to provide visits every 4 hours day and night as would be required. The answer often lies with a syringe-driver. This can be used for diamorphine and to it can be added such drugs as hyoscine, midazolam, or some of the antiemetics, provided the mixture is reconstituted daily. Details of its use and the compatible drugs can be found in chapter 1.

Review whether hyoscine is needed

The 'death rattle' disturbs the relatives, not the patient. No matter how much one explains what it is, and that it is not the patient 'fighting for breath', they are understandably distressed by it. If it is possible to do so, it is better to put the patient onto hyoscine hydrobromide when the first sign of rattle appears. If left until secretions have pooled in the throat, only suction will relieve it.

Hyoscine hydrobromide may be given by subcutaneous injections 0.4 milligram every 4 hours, by syringe-driver 2.4—3.6 milligram over 24 hours, or by transdermal patch placed behind the ear, changed every 72 hours.

A word of caution: given to a conscious patient, hyoscine may produce palpitation and is a frequent cause of mental confusion. If this is experienced, the doctor would be well advised to obtain injection glycopyrrolate, given in a dose of 0.2 milligram every 8 or 12 hours, depending on response. It is equally as effective as hyoscine in relieving secretions but does not produce confusion or psychotic features.

Review medications for emergencies

Pain Always assume that there may be 'incident' or 'breakthrough' pain and plan accordingly. The dose of an opioid for such events should be one-sixth of the total daily opioid intake whether they are on morphine solution every 4 hours or subcutaneous diamorphine by syringe-driver. At home there are several options. Relatives can be told to give additional morphine in exactly the dose that the patient has been getting every 4 hours. Alternatively, they can be taught how to inject diamorphine using one-third of the oral morphine dose, *or* give extra via the syringe-driver by pressing the booster button *for not less than 10 minutes* whilst waiting for a doctor or nurse to come. Clearly, any shorter time will only provide a minuscule dose, totally inadequate for the patient's needs. A syringe-driver is *not* a device for 'patient/relative controlled analgesia' (PCA). If the mouth can be moistened sufficiently, the patient can be given dextromoramide sublingually, remembering that 5 milligram dextromoramide (Palfium) is equivalent to 15 milligram oral morphine, and than even in the final days of life some saliva will be stimulated by a drop of pure lemon juice under the tongue. Naturally, no one would ask a patient to take an extra dose of controlled-release morphine (MST Continus) for breakthrough pain when it takes up to 4 hours to achieve a plasma level. Rather, he should be given an 'immediate-release' morphine preparation.

Convulsions Hopefully the patient now unable to take oral anticonvulsants has already been changed over to intramuscular phenobarbitone or diazepam suppositories. If fits occur, there are three options:

(i)   rectal diazepam solution (Stesolid) 20 milligram, effective within 10–15 minutes (relatives can easily be instructed on its use);
(ii)   subcutaneous midazolam by the nurse (or the relative willing to be instructed on its use and happy to give it; the dose has already been discussed in this text);
(iii)   IV midazolam or Diazemuls given by the doctor as already described.

Restlessness This should not be an inevitable feature of the final days; when it occurs a cause should be sought. Is it pain, a full bladder, or a pressure sore? When no specific treatment is possible, the patient should be given either diazepam suppositories or something added to the syringe-driver such as midazolam, methotrimeprazine, or promazine, preferably the former. This is not an indication for adding haloperidol to the syringe-driver medication.

Haemorrhage If there is any possibility of a massive haemorrhage, the doctor must be prepared to tranquillize the patient using not less than one-third of the day's current requirement of diamorphine and/or midazolam.

Dyspnoea

Terminal dyspnoea, whatever the underlying pathology, does not respond to diuretics alone. What is needed is adequate diamorphine, to which is usefully added midazolam in a dose of one-sixth of the body's previous requirement.

Review the nursing care

Mouth comfort

Candidiasis will continue to be a problem to the end. Nystatin suspension must therefore be continued as part of the care plan. The dying patient, when able to describe his feelings, will speak of his mouth being dry and parched, making speech difficult. The answer is not IV fluids to rehydrate; it is getting the family to offer iced drinks so long as he can take them via a flexi-straw, offering crushed ice cubes (flavoured if so desired) to suck, and showing them how to use lollipop sponges to moisten the mouth of the unconscious patient. They need to be reminded how quickly a mouth becomes dry, particularly if the patient is mouth breathing, and advised to moisten it every 10 minutes.

Pressure part care

The time for frequent turnings has passed! It is now safe and appropriate for the patient to be left almost undisturbed in whatever position is comfortable. Additional padding may be needed for heels, elbows, and knees. Skin care can be less energetic but more time will now need to be spent cooling the skin, sponging and applying talcum powder frequently, and frequently changing the light bedclothes of the patient. If special matresses such as Spenco are needed now, they were needed before and should have been provided!

Bowel care

Energetic bowel care will have been the rule until this stage, but it is no longer a priority. Oral aperients can be stopped and rectal treatment given only if the patient is clearly uncomfortable as a result of a loaded rectum, and not for any other reason.

Bladder care

If the patient is passing little urine, there is no problem now. If he is passing more than a little, it should be discussed whether the patient should be catheterized to save moving him (if male, be fitted with a conveen or a urosheath), or merely kept well padded. Unless the patient strongly objects, catheterization is preferable and strongly to be recommended.

Ambience

Every detail of the sickroom must now be reviewed. Is the bed in the best position for attendants to help the patient? Can the light be dimmed? What arrangements are being made for a night light? Can noise be cut down, ventilation improved, and all extraneous smells be reduced? Are there chairs for the family to sit on, or sleep in, a table for tea cups or mugs, tissues, towels, and pads near at hand?

Review the care of the relatives

Ensure that all are informed and up-to-date

Professionals find it difficult to understand how relatives can say they have not been kept up-to-date, or did not expect the patient to die when it is so obvious that the patient is dying. The fact is that they often do not appreciate that he is at last dying, and research work has repeatedly shown they have not been adequately kept up-to-date by the doctors.

Such research shows that we usually explain the *original* diagnosis and treatment but fail to keep them up-to-date after that. They have known that he is serously ill, and probably that he will die, but that he is actually dying now is a shock. They must be told explicitly, preferably as a family and, better still, with nurse present.

Not only do they need to know that we are talking of the final days, but also *exactly* what will happen in those days. Very likely they have not seen death (except on TV or film and that will hopefully bear no resemblance to a peaceful death at home) or touched a body. The doctor must explain colour changes, cooling of the extremities, Cheyne—Stokes respiration, rattle of secretions, confusion—everything that they may observe and worry about and of which they are possibly too embarrassed and frightened to speak.

Each member of the family (hence the benefit of seeing them all together) needs to be told of the new care plan and priorities: which drugs have been discontinued and why; which are now more important than ever; why and how they will be given; what might happen and the responses the doctor has planned.

It is important to remember that this is not only one of the greatest crises in their life—it is for many a totally new experience for which they feel unprepared and unskilled. They have possibly agreed to care for their loved one at home against great pressure and opposition from friends and relatives. They need every possible professional support. We must never assume that love makes them feel competent to care. Rather the opposite — they may feel that the mark of love is letting the professionals take over.

Enable each relative to help

One well-recognized factor in grief reactions of relatives is the feeling that they were not able, or permitted, to help in the patient's care. At home this need never happen. Anyone can be taught mouth care, sponging and talcing, preparing crushed ice etc. Someone who cannot bear to touch the patient can, for example, do the carrying of drinks up and down stairs, the shopping, or manning the telephone. Some can be taught bladder lavage, others the changing of incontinence pads and, as has been said, a rare few can be instructed in giving injections.

Appropriate care and support of each relative

No family doctor needs to be told how divided families can be and how different is each member. Dying may bring out the best in most patients but it can bring out the worst in the family! Each displays different faces of grief. Some are quiet, others angry. Some ask questions, others pretend they do not want to know. Some suspect the others, but there is nearly always one who either blames the rest or takes command.

The doctor may know many of them. He may elect to speak to each separately but would be wise to get everyone together for an hour or so. He can bring them up-to-date as we have described. He can get them to ask questions and say how each feels about what is happening. He can discern who wants to do what, and who wants permission to withdraw because they cannot cope. It will give him a chance to defuse tension or prevent hostilities, a chance to show how each can contribute and actually grow through this experience.

One or two relatives, particularly the nearest, may benefit from talking about their future and how they see it or fear it. All too often we fail to encourage this expression of anxiety, yet everyone must have it.

Emergency routine

The family may have been telephoning the surgery for years, yet when the patient dies no one can find the telephone number! Worse still, and in the author's view quite unacceptable, they may telephone the doctor only to find none of the partners is on call, and they have to have a deputy come to their loved one.

Prepare a card, written in bold type, and put it beside or behind the telephone in the house. On it write the number where the doctor (or partner) can always be found, where the nurse can be contacted, and the number of their local minister, priest, or rabbi. They should know how and why to contact these people. They do not know how long a person should be kept in pain before calling the doctor and will need to be told. They do not know how bad a fit has to be before calling and must be told. They need to have *everything* explained. It is sad but true. A patient can have the best possible palliation and terminal care at home and the relatives feel pleased that they agreed to it. It only needs an hour or two of pain or dyspnoea or restlessness in the final days for them to forget the weeks which went before and to be left with an indelible memory of 'uncontrolled suffering', for which they will blame themselves and the professional attendants. It need not happen, but much depends on the skills of the primary care team.

10 Grief and bereavement

The members of a primary care team, particularly the doctor, are uniquely placed to help grieving people. They will have been involved with the patient and spouse long before the diagnosis of the life-threatening illness was made, seen them through each of its many stages, and then cared for them in the final weeks and months. Hopefully the doctor will continue as the adviser of the bereaved spouse or close family for years to come. The honour and the responsibility are considerable.

In this area, the roles of doctor and nurse are different but complementary. The nurse will spend longer in the home with them and often become almost one of the family, getting to know and understand a different side of them. Unlike the doctor, however, the nurse may not have seen the family at times of health, and after the terminally ill patient has died may not have other reasons to revisit that home. If the practice has a social worker, he or she may also have become involved, partly to assist with special benefits and financial arrangements, and also hopefully in showing the family how to use their undoubted strengths to cope with many frightening changes in their lives. If there is a Church connection, the clergyman will also have become involved but, sadly, fewer and fewer families have such a connection. It must be almost as difficult for the clergyman to be called in to a strange family at such a crisis as it is for a deputizing doctor to an emergency house call!

GRIEF

There are some things about grief which, although they may appear self-evident, bear repetition.

Grief starts when the diagnosis is made

It might even be said that grieving starts *before* the diagnosis is made, when the patient is clearly unwell and being urged to see the doctor, when the loved one senses that there is something seriously wrong. When the diagnosis is suspected, or finally made, no matter how optimistic an outlook is given, most relatives fear the worst but may not mention those fears or grief to anyone. Often it is only after the death that they admit to having silently grieved over what they always feared would happen.

Their silent grieving may be made more difficult if, for some reason, the patient has not been honestly informed of the diagnosis but the relatives are aware of it. Perhaps, as so often happens, they have vetoed the patient being told or, again as so frequently occurs, were told of the diagnosis in considerable detail but not thereafter kept up-to-date with developments.

Cancer brings its own unique problems. With modern treatment, patients go into long spells of remission with high hopes of cure, only to have them dashed during each relapse. The confidence of the surgeon who reported taking 'most of it away' is conveyed to relatives, who understandably wonder what happens to the portion he left behind. Hopes rise each time the patient sees another specialist who seems so positive about what he can offer with radiotherapy or chemotherapy, but the relatives (like the patient) cannot fail to notice how each remission is shorter than the previous one, each relapse more dramatic. Experience shows that by this time the eventual outcome is well recognized by the patient and relatives, but they increasingly keep their feelings to themselves, each wrapped up in their own grief, each fearing that talking it through with each other would only hurt the ones they love. So grief deepens, made worse by partial knowledge, a conspiracy of silence, and secret questions and feelings hidden from the world.

Grief is not always physiological

There are still doctors who speak of all grief and sadness as 'physiological', something we must all bear, and for which we are all equipped. Even if, as all would agree, loss is a feature of life and will be experienced in many forms at different times by each of us, we can all be comforted and supported. This is a role of the family doctor. By so doing, he or she is not 'making a mountain out of a molehill', not medicalizing a physiological reaction. He is acting as a friend and caring fellow human being, better able to help than most others because his knowledge and communication skills enable him to replace fear with knowledge.

Grief carries a definite morbidity

It is widely accepted that widowers have a much higher risk of developing a serious illness in the first year of their bereavement. Many others report more episodes of illness when they are grieving than might otherwise be the case. If any of these can be prevented or mitigated, the family doctor is well placed to do so.

Grief can be predicted

Some guidelines will be given in this chapter to help in forecasting how some people will react and who may be at particular risk. Once again we see the challenge of good palliative care: planning and anticipation as far as is possible.

Grief can change individuals and families

No one is ever the same again after they have lost a loved one. Every doctor can recall the irresponsible teenager who seemed to grow up and mature as a result, just as he can recount tales of families torn asunder because they could not cope. Some people turn to alcohol or drugs, but many more become more mature and responsible. Death is not always an unwelcome blow. Some find much wanted freedom after years of unhappy marriage, others relish the chance to take up new posts, pursue old ambitions, or study for further qualifications, displaying previously dormant gifts. Just as dying patients often discover their real selves at the end of life, so do many bereaved people who then go on into another phase of life. Not all change is destructive, but we sometimes overlook this in our society, which often seeks to deny the creative powers which can be unleashed as a result of loss, whether by death or disability.

FACTORS AFFECTING GRIEF OUTCOME

Time to prepare for the deceased's death

We all know that the most devastating loss is the unexpected one, for example, the sudden death from a myocardial infarction or a road traffic accident. When someone can be helped to come to terms with an expected death, there will still be deep sadness but it will usually not be either so prolonged or so destructive if they were supported, kept informed, and shown how to share in the care.

It must not be assumed that, the longer a person knows that the death of a loved one is inevitable, the easier it will be. Paradoxically, a very protracted death can also produce bereavement problems if it lasted much longer than expected, certainly longer than the relatives had subconsciously programmed themselves for. When someone has sat at a bedside day in and day out for months or years, no matter how prepared they may be for the death, the change in the pattern of daily living afterwards can lead to problems.

The long, terminal phase may be a feature of the disease process whether from cardiac, neurological, or degenerative conditions, but a somewhat different problem can be produced by modern cancer management. Many cancer patients go in and out of genuine remissions or, to the relatives, look as though they are going to die and then improve remarkably as a result of their radiotherapy, chemotherapy, or even palliative medicine or surgery. Such happy outcomes may have been expected by the doctors, but do we often enough appreciate how baffling and sometimes unnerving they can be for relatives? They have been told that the disease was incurable, yet time after time the patient improves, only to relapse again. It is easy to see why some relatives think that the doctors, in spite of what they have said, are actually aiming to cure, or at least to gain time until a cure is found.

Opportunity to care for the patient

If only more people appreciated the importance of this when, for what they regard as good reason, they press for their loved one to be admitted to a hospital or hospice. Providing they themselves are cared for, and their own needs recognized, people can actually benefit from having shared in the physical care of the loved one.

In these days of institutionalized medical care, it may not be easy to persuade relatives of this, but it is one reason for publishing this book. Immediate relatives could do much more nursing care than they are currently allowed, or encouraged, to do, at home or in hospital. One of the topics for regular review in the primary care team meetings should be the caring done by family, what more they could do, who should instruct and guide them, and how they should be encouraged and supported in doing it.

Relatives' perception of support

Those who do not *feel* supported or understood often suffer bad grief reactions, irrespective of how much help they may in fact have received. We have all met such people. It should be noted that they are not necessarily unaware or unappreciative of the support given to the patient, but of the help given to them, the carers. 'Oh yes, doctor visited regularly and certainly looked after John, but what did he ever do for me? Come to think of it, what did anyone do for me at any time!'

It is important to appreciate that we are not speaking of that partial amnesia which so often occurs immediately after a death. We are speaking of people who, months or even years later, speak as if no doctor, nurse, clergyman, neighbour, or friend ever once spoke to them or offered to help, when it is known that this is not the case.

Unresolved previous grief

Someone who has not yet 'got over' a bereavement of a year or two before is at risk. Perhaps it is still so recent; perhaps they simply needed longer to recover; perhaps they needed help and no one has recognized this. Whatever the reason, the family doctor may be well placed to know of other losses and appreciate the added burden the new one will bring. Some people only begin to grieve for the previous loss when they start to grieve for the latest one.

Poor relationship with the deceased

It has already been said that not everyone regards death as a disaster. For some it may be a release, a new freedom. For many others it can be a reminder of a relationship which could have been better had both parties worked harder at it—now that opportunity has passed for ever. They suffer a form of guilt reaction which may surprise even the family doctor, who has so often witnessed the bitterness and mutual blame over many years. The widow who has rarely had a good word to say about her husband may suffer a profound grief reaction and begin to speak as if their relationship had been blissful.

Poor socioeconomic circumstances

In bereavement, as in so many clinical conditions, people from poor socio-economic circumstances often fare badly.

FEATURES OF NORMAL GRIEF

It might be thought that these are so well known that there is nothing more to add. There are, however, some features of which even the professionals may be unaware and it is only these which will be described here.

A surprisingly large percentage of grievers experience some of the same symptoms as did the one who has died. The widow of a cardiac patient may suffer palpitations, dyspnoea or chest tightness; that of the man who died of a gastric carcinoma may experience dyspepsia or epigastric fullness, and so on. Seldom will they report these symptoms, however, in case they are labelled as neurotic or become a 'nuisance' to the doctor.

Even more grievers experience what might be termed hallucinations although they have no other features of psychiatric illness. The widower is sure he heard his wife say, as she had done hundreds of times in their life together, that she was going upstairs to bed and that he should lock the door. The widow is sure she can smell his pipe or his aftershave. Others report the poignancy of sensing the loved one in bed beside them and reaching over to find cold emptiness. Again, these experiences may not be reported. The possibility of them occurring needs to be mentioned, with the strongest possible reassurance that they are all normal and not features of incipient physical or psychiatric illness.

FEATURES OF ABNORMAL GRIEF

Members of a primary care team should be alert to the following features, the occurrence of even one or two of which should raise their concern for that patient and challenge them to ask what is to be done and by whom:

(1) when the griever is known to have a serious personality disorder, a history of depressive illness, or of suicidal ideation;

(2) when the griever repeatedly speaks of suicide or persists with an attitude of hopelessness or low self-esteem;
(3) when someone, months after the death, continues to feel unsupported and ignored through the illness and subsequent bereavement in spite of all the evidence to the contrary;
(4) when 'progress' stops and the griever regresses—they had begun to mix with others, had taken up some social activities, and looked as though they were winning through, when it all stopped and they became reclusive and uncommunicative;
(5) when increasingly frequent consultations with the family doctor reveal no serious organic disease and all emotional distress is denied;
(6) when there is increasing resort to alcohol, tranquillizers, or hypnotics, particularly when they are not being prescribed by the doctor.

If the doctor feels competent to handle such problems, this is all well and good. These problems are not easy to handle, are usually time-consuming, and failure may result in suicide, parasuicide, or prolonged depressive illness and social isolation. Often the best course is to seek psychiatric help or to enquire whether the local branch of a bereavement counselling agency (in Britain: CRUSE) would feel competent to help.

Whatever action is taken, *each* member of the primary care team must be alerted to the problem and appraised of the care plan, with a detailed report put in the case notes.

STAGES OF GRIEF

Relief

This is particularly seen after a chronic death and rarely after a sudden, unexpected one. It usually lasts for a few days and is characterized by happiness for the deceased ('Thank goodness he'll not have any more suffering') coupled with personal relief ('I couldn't have coped for much longer'). There is much gratitude expressed to care-givers and a pervading sense of unreality and numbness ('I can't take it all in, I simply can't believe that he's gone').

The numbness and slight amnesia may worry the carers. They may forget usually well-remembered addresses and telephone numbers, the name of the clergyman, or advice so recently given by the professionals. Curiously, months and years later, they will probably be able to recall what may seem to be the most trivial details, such as what the doctor was wearing, or what a neighbour said.

This is not the time for a doctor to be advising or counselling, and certainly not the time for tranquillizers, antidepressants, or hypnotics, though well-meaning family and friends often expect the doctor to offer the latter.

Relaxation

This follows the funeral and lasts until family members have to go their separate ways. This may not be long, but there is a sense of family unity and shared pain. Differences are often temporarily forgotten and time is spent reminiscing and doing the many practical things which can be so demanding and worrying.

While relatives and friends are there to support the family, the doctor need only visit occasionally, more as a mark of friendship than for professional reasons. As the time for them to go approaches, he must ensure that arrangements are in place for regular contact, that no precipitate decisions are being made for moving house, getting rid of the patient's clothes and possessions, burning letters, and destroying trophies. It can be reassuring for family members to see the practical concern of a doctor at this time before they leave the family home.

Resentment

The family have gone home and life has returned to normal for everyone— except the griever! For him or her there is a profound sense not only of loneliness and unreality, but also 'aloneness'. They feel disbelief, self-pity, and soon find themselves criticizing self, family, and professional carers, the same people who only weeks before had done no wrong. Every detail of the loved one's illness and care is gone over again and again, often accompanied by doubts of the appropriateness of care and the attitude and actions of others.

Their increasing pain, self-doubt, and loss of purpose in life are in contrast to their healthy appearance, often remarked on by others, and the frequency with which they experience the symptoms and hallucinations already mentioned.

Many later recall that one of the worst times was the *three-month mark*. Friends stopped asking about their health, preferring to exclaim how well they looked; rather than mentioning the loved one, they began to cross to the other side of the street to avoid embarrassing encounters. Particularly painful is the frequency with which friends speak of their holidays or plans, insensitively forgetting that, for the griever, there can only be unfulfilled dreams.

The doctor can do much by repeating again and again how prolonged and painful normal grief can be, why caring friends behave as they do, and reassuring by all means possible that the griever is well and fully deserving of the doctor's attention.

Remembrance

Starting after about three months and often continuing well past the first painful anniversary, this period is characterized by a slow return to normal activities and the gradual taking-up of some modest social life. Outwardly they look well but the slightest thing can trigger tears or waves of loneliness, self-pity, and recriminations.

It is worth remembering that the time when most suicide attempts are made in bereavement is seven months after the death, sometimes after veiled threats to do so, but often when the person otherwise *appears* to be recovering well.

Repair

At last, often 15–24 months after the death, the griever clearly and consciously begins to rebuild his or her life. New interests are developed, careers pursued, new hobbies and sports started. It must never be forgotten, however, that there will always be anniversaries almost too painful to bear yet often apparently overlooked even by family and friends—Christmas, a birthday, a wedding anniversary, and each anniversary of the death.

BEREAVEMENT SUPPORT BY THE DOCTOR

The following guidelines are suggested:

1. Remember the pattern of bereavement and respond accordingly.
2. Remember the risk factors for abnormal grief and try to identify (with the help of primary care team colleagues) those who may need closer watching and support.
3. Remember the features of abnormal grief and be on the alert so that immediate skilled care can be given.
4. Remember the therapeutic benefits of firm and informed reassurance and thorough clinical examination for those fearing the development of their own fatal illness.
5. Keep a diary of patient deaths and try to pay an informal home visit around the first anniversary. Contrary to what some might think, it will not be many because some deaths will have been of those without local relatives or the grievers may themselves have since died.
6. Do not expect grievers to come to the doctor of their own accord but rather invite them, explaining how keen you are to see them come through it, and give them an appointment.
7. Get to know the local bereavement counselling service and use them. Research shows that for most clients such trained volunteers are as useful as the professionals.
8. Do not rush into prescribing. Inability to sleep is normal in early bereavement and not likely to be much helped by benzodiazepines. If it is thought essential to prescribe them, make sure it is for a strictly limited time. Grief may be intensely painful and depressing but routine antidepressants will not help. The best prescription, as so often in good primary care, is a sensitive, sensible doctor.

Appendix 1: Setting up a syringe-driver (Graseby Medical — Model MS16A) to deliver a 24-hour subcutaneous infusion of diamorphine

1. Syringe-driver speed is set at 2 mm per hour.
2. 10 ml of sterile water is drawn up in a 10 ml syringe.
3. The required amount of diamorphine for the 24-hour period is dissolved in 1−2 ml of the water from the syringe and then drawn up.
4. The syringe is attached to the syringe-driver, making sure that the plunger and pump are in contact.
5. The butterfly needle is inserted subcutaneously in the anterior abdominal wall, upper chest wall, or over the insertion of deltoid, and held in place with adhesive film such as Tegaderm or Micropore tape (3M Health Care).
6. The syringe-driver battery is inserted and the starter button pressed; in the first 24 hours, the function of the driver should be checked every 6 hours.
7. The site of infusion should be changed every 3 or 4 days.
8. If adequate analgesia is not achieved:

    • check the syringe-driver and battery
    • check the infusion set connections for leaks
    • check the infusion site for signs of local irritation.

Appendix 2: Using a TENS (transcutaneous electrical nerve stimulator)

1. Connect electrodes to TENS.
2. Apply electrode jelly to paddles.
3. Place one paddle over spinal processes two dermatomes above affected dermatomes and affix firmly using strong, non-allergenic surgical adhesive tape.
4. Place the other 'migrating' paddle over the worst area of pain and again affix securely.
5. Switch on TENS, starting at lowest voltage and lowest frequency.
6. Slowly increase voltage until patient describes 'tingling' feelings; if this does not occur at highest voltage, slowly increase the frequency until it does.
7. At the point of 'tingling', minimally reduce frequency and voltage until sensation stops and wait 5–10 minutes.
8. Slowly increase the frequency and voltage to the point where 'tingling' occurred and if it no longer happens, prescribe that as the recommended dose.
9. Leave *in situ* for 48 hours, except for checking there is adequate electrode jelly.
10. After 48 hours of continuous use, the routine should be 4 hours on, 4 hours off etc., until no pain is experienced.
11. As the site of pain moves, the spinal electrode should be kept in place and the migrating electrode moved appropriately to the site of pain.

Appendix 3: Electrode positions commonly used for TENS

a) Anterior aspect
b) Posterior aspect

(Reproduced with permission from *Oxford Textbook of Palliative Medicine*)

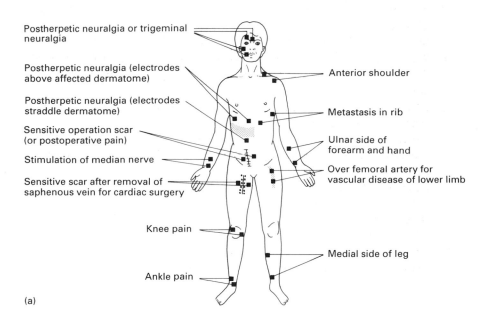

Postherpetic neuralgia or trigeminal neuralgia

Postherpetic neuralgia (electrodes above affected dermatome)

Postherpetic neuralgia (electrodes straddle dermatome)

Sensitive operation scar (or postoperative pain)

Stimulation of median nerve

Sensitive scar after removal of saphenous vein for cardiac surgery

Knee pain

Ankle pain

Anterior shoulder

Metastasis in rib

Ulnar side of forearm and hand

Over femoral artery for vascular disease of lower limb

Medial side of leg

(a)

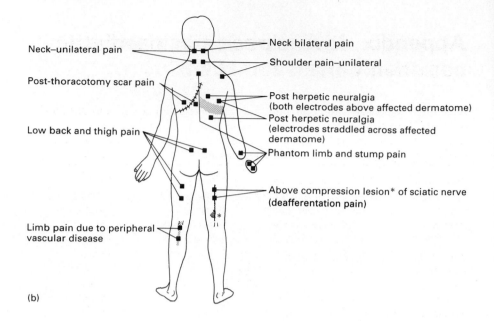

Neck–unilateral pain

Neck bilateral pain

Shoulder pain–unilateral

Post-thoracotomy scar pain

Post herpetic neuralgia
(both electrodes above affected dermatome)

Post herpetic neuralgia
(electrodes straddled across affected
dermatome)

Low back and thigh pain

Phantom limb and stump pain

Above compression lesion* of sciatic nerve
(deafferentation pain)

Limb pain due to peripheral
vascular disease

(b)

Appendix 4: Analgesics in paediatric palliative care

Recommended dosages of commonly used analgesics and adjuncts in paediatric palliative care patients.

Medication	Dose and frequency		Route
Paracetamol	10–15 milligram/kg	4-hourly	Oral
	15–20 milligram/kg	4-hourly	Rectal
Aspirin	10–15 milligram/kg	4-hourly	Oral
Ibuprofen	4–10 milligram/kg	6–8-hourly	Oral
Tolmetin	5–7 milligram/kg	6–8-hourly	Oral
Naproxen	5–10 milligram/kg	8–12-hourly	Oral
Morphine	0.15–0.3 milligram/kg	2–4-hourly	Oral/rectal
sulphate[a]	0.05–0.1 milligram/kg	2–4-hourly	IV/SC
	0.01–0.04 milligram/kg	1-hourly	IV/SC infusion
Sustained-release morphine	0.3–0.6 milligram/kg	12-hourly	Oral
Codeine	0.5–1.0 milligram/kg	3–4-hourly	Oral
Imipramine	0.2 milligram/kg[b]	Every hour of sleep	Oral

[a] There is no ceiling dose for morphine; the dose should be adjusted according to the patient's requirements.

[b] May be increased to 3 milligram/kg every hour of sleep over 2–3 weeks.

(Reproduced with permission from *Oxford Textbook of Palliative Medicine*)

Appendix 5: Pain chart using a visual analogue scale

Patient's name: _____

Reference number/Date of birth: _____

PAIN REPORT

DATE   8 a.m.   8 p.m.

	NO PAIN	UNBEARABLE PAIN		NO PAIN	UNBEARABLE PAIN
___	.___.___.___.___.			.___.___.___.___.	
___	.___.___.___.___.			.___.___.___.___.	
___	.___.___.___.___.			.___.___.___.___.	
___	.___.___.___.___.			.___.___.___.___.	
___	.___.___.___.___.			.___.___.___.___.	
___	.___.___.___.___.			.___.___.___.___.	
___	.___.___.___.___.			.___.___.___.___.	

NOTE: 1. This record should be completed by the patient, not the family.
        2. The report should be left out for doctor and sister to see.

Appendix 6: Recording nausea using a visual analogue scale

Patient's name: _____

Reference number/Date of birth: _____

NAUSEA REPORT

DATE   8 a.m.   8 p.m.

NO NAUSEA	UNBEARABLE NAUSEA		NO NAUSEA	UNBEARABLE NAUSEA

NO NAUSEA   UNBEARABLE NAUSEA   NO NAUSEA   UNBEARABLE NAUSEA

NO NAUSEA   UNBEARABLE NAUSEA   NO NAUSEA   UNBEARABLE NAUSEA

NO NAUSEA   UNBEARABLE NAUSEA   NO NAUSEA   UNBEARABLE NAUSEA

NO NAUSEA   UNBEARABLE NAUSEA   NO NAUSEA   UNBEARABLE NAUSEA

NO NAUSEA   UNBEARABLE NAUSEA   NO NAUSEA   UNBEARABLE NAUSEA

NO NAUSEA   UNBEARABLE NAUSEA   NO NAUSEA   UNBEARABLE NAUSEA

NO NAUSEA   UNBEARABLE NAUSEA   NO NAUSEA   UNBEARABLE NAUSEA

NOTE: 1. This record should be completed by the patient, not the family.
2. The report should be left out for doctor and sister to see.

Appendix 7: Recording breathlessness using a visual analogue scale

Patient's name: _____

Reference number/Date of birth: _____

BREATHLESSNESS REPORT

DATE   8 a.m.   8 p.m.

NO BREATHLESSNESS	UNBEARABLE BREATHLESSNESS	NO BREATHLESSNESS	UNBEARABLE BREATHLESSNESS

(repeated seven times, for both 8 a.m. and 8 p.m. columns)

NO BREATHLESSNESS — UNBEARABLE BREATHLESSNESS
·____·____·____·____·____·

NO BREATHLESSNESS — UNBEARABLE BREATHLESSNESS
·____·____·____·____·____·

NO BREATHLESSNESS — UNBEARABLE BREATHLESSNESS
·____·____·____·____·____·

NO BREATHLESSNESS — UNBEARABLE BREATHLESSNESS
·____·____·____·____·____·

NO BREATHLESSNESS — UNBEARABLE BREATHLESSNESS
·____·____·____·____·____·

NO BREATHLESSNESS — UNBEARABLE BREATHLESSNESS
·____·____·____·____·____·

NO BREATHLESSNESS — UNBEARABLE BREATHLESSNESS
·____·____·____·____·____·

NOTE: 1. This record should be completed by the patient, not the family.
2. The report should be left out for doctor and sister to see.

Appendix 8: Suggested chart for recording medication

NAME JOHN SMITH	COMMUNITY NURSING SISTER					M. BROWN			
	am	am	pm	pm	pm	am			
NAME OF DRUG	6	10	2	6	10	2			
Metoclopramide 10 mg	✓		✓		✓				
Dexamethasone 2 mg		✓							
Morphine solution 10 ml	✓	✓	✓	✓	✓	✓			
Temazepam 10 mg					✓				
Piroxicam 10 mg		✓							

Family Practice Name and Address   Tel. No.

Appendix 9: Drugs and equipment for the doctor's bag

The contents of a family doctor's bag are often a reflection of his personality and practice and, sadly, must now take into account the increasing attention paid by drug addicts and criminals to some of the contents. The suggestions made here are drugs and preparations of particular value in domiciliary palliative care, particularly for the emergencies already discussed.

DIAMORPHINE 30 MILLIGRAM AMPOULES

Most, but by no means all, patients on opioids will be on doses less than 30 milligram every 4 hours (i.e. equivalent to oral morphine 90 milligram). This dose will therefore be adequate for such emergencies as haemorrhage, vertebral collapse, pathological fractures, and incident pain, particularly in hepatic secondaries.

There is little to be said for the popular combined preparation of morphine and cyclizine (Cyclimorph) where the opioid dose is small and the unnecessary antiemetic has a propensity for producing sedation and confusion, particularly in the elderly.

DEXAMETHASONE INJECTION
(4 MILLIGRAM PER ML IN 2 ML AMPOULES)

Two ampoules should be carried, i.e. 16 milligram in all, adequate for SVC obstruction, spinal cord compression, and acute cerebral oedema. Though severe hypercalcaemia will require hospitalization for saline rehydration and pamidronate, intravenous dexamethasone occasionally helps in the less severe cases whilst awaiting emergency calcium and albumin biochemistry results.

HYOSCINE HYDROBROMIDE
(400 MILLIGRAM PER AMPOULE)

Though, as described, this should preferably be given every 4 hours or as a subcutaneous infusion via a syringe-driver, it can be given as an emergency to reduce the 'death rattle' pending the more leisurely setting up of the driver.

HYOSCINE BUTYLBROMIDE
(BUSCOPAN 20 MILLIGRAM PER AMPOULE)

A valuable antispasmodic, this drug can be used for the pain of subacute obstruction, colic of any type, acute cholangitis, and bladder spasm.

MIDAZOLAM INJECTION (5 MILLIGRAM PER ML)

This is one of the most useful drugs in domiciliary palliative care, particularly because of its rapid onset of action, useful as an emergency tranquillizer for panic attacks, in extreme agitation (provided it is not caused by pain where an appropriate analgesic is needed), and as an anticonvulsant.

The dose range is 1.25–125 milligram depending on the size and age of the patient ('the younger the patient the higher the dose'), and whether or not the patient is a regular benzodiazepine-taker, making a higher dose necessary.

It should usually be given subcutaneously but can be given intravenously provided the injection rate does not exceed 1 milligram per minute. Its ability to depress respiration must be remembered particularly when administered intravenously. Because of its short half-life, benefit may last no longer than 3 hours.

DIAZEPAM INJECTION
(DIAZEMULS 10 MILLIGRAM PER AMPOULE)

Given only by intravenous injection at a rate of 1 milligram per minute, this benzodiazepine has the same uses as midazolam, but has metabolites with a much longer half-life and consequently more protracted sedation.

DIAZEPAM RECTAL SOLUTION
(STESOLID 10 MILLIGRAM PER TUBE)

Easily administered rectally via its lubricated nozzle, a therapeutic effect is evident within 15 minutes, making it useful when IV administration is not necessary or difficult, and for administration by lay carers instructed in its use.

HALOPERIDOL INJECTION

In doses as small as 1.25 milligram or 2.5 milligram subcutaneously, this is one of the best antiemetics, particularly for opioid-induced nausea and vomiting.

When used for acute paranoid psychotic episodes, it needs to be given intravenously in doses as high as 5 milligram and 10 milligram until the patient has been sedated. It should be remembered that haloperidol has a long half-life, producing sedation lasting several days.

METHOTRIMEPRAZINE INJECTION (NOZINAN)

This little-used phenothiazine is valuable as a major tranquillizer, antiemetic, antipruritic, antihiccup drug with a modest analgesic effect. It is given in emergencies by intramuscular injection in doses of 25—50 milligram, repeated if necessary every 4 hours.

In most respects similar to chlorpromazine (Largactil), methotrimeprazine is *much* more sedative. Experience suggests that it is a valuable drug when given on a regular basis but, for emergency sedation, it is not preferable to midazolam.

LIGNOCAINE 2 PER CENT INJECTION

There will be occasions when a patient with, for example, pathological rib fractures or sudden exquisite pain in a skin metastasis will be best helped not with a systemic analgesic but with a local infiltration of 2 per cent lignocaine.

It is presumed that every doctor will carry the following in his bag: injectable metoclopramide and frusemide, a urinary catheter, anaesthetic jelly, and a catheter pack.

Appendix 10: Useful organizations

Age Concern

England:
60 Pitcairn Road
Mitcham
Surrey CR4 3LL
tel. 081 640 5431

Scotland:
54A Fountainbridge
Edinburgh
EH3 9PT
tel. 031 288 5656

Alzheimer's Disease Society

England:
158/160 Balham High Road
London
tel. 071 675 6557

Scotland:
33 Castle Street
Edinburgh
tel. 031 225 1453

ACT (Action for the Care of Families whose children have life-threatening and terminal conditions)
Institute of Child Health, Royal Hospital for Sick Children, St Michael's Hill, Bristol BS2 8BJ, tel. 0272 221556. Parents and professionals may either telephone or write for information about support services and self-help groups, including children's hospices.

Association of Crossroads Care Attendant Schemes
10 Regent Place, Rugby, Warwickshire, CV21 2PN, tel. 0788 573653. This organization provides care attendants who come into the home to provide a break for the carers. Applications should be made either to the above address or to:

Scotland:
24 George Square
Glasgow G2 1EG
tel. 041 226 3793

North Wales:
Crossroads
The North Wales Regional Office
104–106 High Street
Mold
Clwyd CH7 1VH
tel. 0352 750544

South Wales (Main Office):
Crossroads Wales
5 Coopers Yard
Trade Street
Cardiff
CF1 5DF
tel. 0222 222282

BACUP
3 Bath Place, Rivington Street, London EC2A 3JR, tel. 071 613 2121; free-phone outside London: 0800 181 199. This organization helps patients and their families cope with cancer. You may either telephone or write and specially-trained cancer nurses will provide information, support, and practical advice. In addition, the organization publishes many useful leaflets and booklets on different forms of cancer and their treatment.

Breast Care and Mastectomy Association for Great Britain
15/19 Britten Street, London SW3 3TZ, helpline telephone number: 071 867 1103.

Scotland:

Suite 2/8
65 Bath Street
Glasgow G2 2PS
tel. 041 353 1050

13A Castle Terrace
Edinburgh EH1 2DP
tel. 031 221 0407

This organization, partly staffed by volunteers who have themselves had breast cancer, offers practical advice, information, and support to women concerned about breast cancer.

British Colostomy Association
15 Station Road, Reading, Berkshire RG1 1LG, tel. 0734 391537. This is an information and advisory service, partly staffed by helpers who have themselves long experience of living with a colostomy, offering information, reassurance, and encouragement to patients with colostomies.

British Red Cross Society
9 Grosvenor Crescent, London SW1X 7EJ, tel. 071 235 5454. (Local offices are listed in telephone directories and Yellow Pages.) The British Red Cross offers a range of services of use to cancer patients, including the loan of wheelchairs and other pieces of equipment.

Cancerlink
17 Britannia Street, London WC1X 9JN; tel. 071 833 2451. This organization provides emotional support and information on all aspects of cancer to help patients, families, and friends and also acts as a coordinating resource for cancer support and self-help groups throughout the country. Enquirers in Scotland should contact Cancerlink Scotland, 9 Castle Terrace, Edinburgh EH1 2DP, tel. 031 228 5557.

Cancer Relief Macmillan Fund
15/19 Britten Street, London SW3 3TZ, tel. 071 352 7811. Enquirers in Scotland should contact the Scottish office at: 9 Castle Terrace, Edinburgh EH1 2DP, tel. 031 228 5557. This major national charity helps patients and their families in many ways. It pump-primes the establishment of Macmillan Nursing Services, does much to encourage professional education in cancer care, and has a patient grants department, providing financial help towards the cost of a wide range of needs for people with cancer. Applications for such grants are usually made by a Home Care Nurse, a Health Visitor or Community Nurse, or by a Social Worker.

Carer's National Association

England:	Scotland:
22 Chilworth Mews	11 Queen's Crescent
London W2 3RG	Glasgow G4 9AS
tel. 071 724 7776	tel. 041 333 9495

This organization provides information and support for people caring for patients at home and has a range of free leaflets.

Chest, Heart and Stroke Association
65 North Castle Street, Edinburgh EH2 3LT, tel. 031 225 6963.

Compassionate Friends
6 Denmark Street, Bristol BS1 5DQ, tel. 0272 292778. This is a befriending rather than a counselling service for parents whose child of any age has died from whatever cause. Information can be provided about local groups nation-wide.

CRUSE Bereavement Care
Cruse House, 126 Sheen Road, Richmond, Surrey TW9 1UR, tel. 081 940 4818.

Scotland:	Wales:
18 South Trinity Road	Bryn Tirion, Churchill Close
Edinburgh EH5 3PN	Llanblethian
tel. 031 551 1511	Cowbridge
	South Glamorgan CF7 7JH
	tel. 0446 775351.

This national organization for bereavement care and counselling now has more than 200 branches throughout the United Kingdom, their addresses and tele-phone numbers to be found in the directory or Yellow Pages. Those in need may make direct approach to a local branch or be referred or recommended by family doctor, Health Visitor, Macmillan Nurse, or friends. Most branches offer one-to-one counselling either in the office or the person's home, plus social groups, children's counselling, and social activities.

Foundation for Black Bereaved Families
11 Kingston Square, Salter's Hill, London SE19 1JE, tel. 081 761 7228. The Foundation offers counselling, financial advice and support for bereaved black people of Afro-Caribbean origin.

Gay Bereavement Project
Unitarium Rooms, Hope Lane, London NW11 8BS, tel. 081 455 8894. This is a telephone helpline service for people bereaved by the death of a partner of the same sex.

Graseby Medical Ltd
Colonial Way, Watford WD2 4LJ, tel. 09232 46434. (The manufacturers and suppliers of syringe-drivers.)

Help The Aged
England:
  16/18 St James' Walk
  London
  EC1R 0BE
  tel. 071 253 0253

Scotland:
  53 Blackfriars Street
  Edinburgh
  EH1 1NB
  tel. 031 556 4666

Hodgkin's Disease Association
PO Box 275, Haddenham, Aylesbury, Buckinghamshire HP17 8JJ, tel. 0844 291500. As this name implies, this organization offers information and emotional support for patients suffering from both Hodgkin's Disease and non-Hodgkin's Lymphoma, as well as their families.

Hospice Information Service
St Christopher's Hospice, 51–59 Lawrie Park Road, Sydenham, London SE26 6DZ, tel. 081 778 9252. This service publishes an invaluable Directory of Hospice Services in the United Kingdom and Ireland, including basic details of hospices, Home Care Teams, and Hospital Support Teams.

Irish Cancer Society
5 Northumberland Road, Dublin 4, Republic of Ireland, tel. 010 3531 681855 (Freephone in Eire 1800 200300). The freephone service offers information on all aspects of cancer from specially trained nurses. The Society funds home care and rehabilitation programmes, offers support groups and, on the request of the patient's doctor or public health nurse, a home night nursing service.

Leukaemia Care Society
PO Box 82, Exeter EH2 5DP, tel. 0392 64848. This Society promotes the welfare of patients and their families suffering from leukaemia and allied blood disorders, offering support, friendship, information leaflets, and financial assistance.

Malcolm Sargent Cancer Fund for Children
14 Abingdon Road, London W8 6AF, tel. 071 936 4548. This organization is for young people under the age of 21 who have any form of cancer, whether they are in hospital or in their own home.

Marie Curie Cancer Care
28 Belgrave Square, London SW1X 8QG, tel. 071 235 3325. This is another major charity which not only runs several large hospices but also funds home nursing services and is active in professional education and cancer research.

National Association of Laryngectomy Clubs
Ground Floor, 6 Ricket Street, London SW6 1RU, tel. 071 381 9993. This Association encourages rehabilitation, speech therapy, social support and advises on special aids and equipment for laryngectomees.

National Holiday Fund for Sick and Disabled Children
Suite 1, Princess House, 1–2 Princess Parade, New Road, Dagenham, Essex RM10 9LS, tel. 081 595 9624. This Fund provides holidays throughout the world for children between 8 and 18 years of age with either chronic or terminal conditions.

Stroke Association
CHSA House, Whitecross Street, London EC1Y 8JJ, tel. 071 490 7999.

Tak Tent
G Block, Western Infirmary, Dumbarton Road, Glasgow G11 6NT, tel. 041 332 2639. This organization, which started in Glasgow, has now spawned groups throughout Scotland, offering emotional support, counselling, and information on cancers and treatments, as well as running various 'Coping with Cancer' courses.

Appendix 11: Bibliography

Doyle, D., Hanks, G. W., and MacDonald, N. (Eds) (1993). *Oxford textbook of palliative medicine*. Oxford University Press, Oxford.
(This is the definitive reference text on all aspects of palliative care—pain and symptom control in adults and children, psychological problems, spiritual, ethical and cultural issues, domiciliary care, AIDS, neurological and endocrine problems etc.)

CLINICAL AND THERAPEUTIC

Cochrane, G. M. (1987). *The management of motor neurone disease*. Churchill Livingstone, Edinburgh.

Saunders, C. (1993). *The management of terminal malignant disease*. Edward Arnold, London.

Scottish Health Education Group (1989). *Coping with dementia*. Scottish Health Education Group, Edinburgh. (Written for the lay carer but of value to the professionals.)

Twycross, R. G. and Lack, S. (1983). *Symptom control in far-advanced cancer: pain relief*. Pitman, London.

Twycross, R. G. and Lack, S. (1986). *Control of alimentary symptoms in far-advanced cancer*. Churchill Livingstone, Edinburgh.

Twycross, R. G. and Lack, S. (1990). *Therapeutics in terminal cancer*. Churchill Livingstone, London.

COMMUNICATION

Buckman, R. (1988). *I don't know what to say—how to help and support someone who is dying*. Macmillan, London. (A book of inestimable value to professionals and lay carers).

Buckman, R. (1993). *How to break bad news—a guide for healthcare professionals*. Macmillan Medical, London. (Easy to read, making it all seem like common sense.)

Lichter, I. (1987). *Communication in cancer care*. Churchill Livingstone, Edinburgh. (A book of common sense, wisdom, and sensitivity written by a retired thoracic surgeon.)

Stedeford, A. (1994). *Facing death: patients, families, and professionals.* Second edition. Sobell Publications, Oxford. (A helpful book for professionals and caring relatives on the emotional problems and needs of all concerned, written by a psychiatrist experienced in palliative care.)

GRIEF AND BEREAVEMENT

Hinton, J. (1972). *Dying.* Penguin Books, London. (A useful book on grief and bereavement written by a psychiatrist associated with St Christopher's Hospice, London.)

Kopp, R. (1947). *When someone you love is dying: a handbook for counsellors and those who care.* Zondervan Publishing House, Grand Rapids, Michigan. (Practical and encouraging.)

Parkes, C. M. (1986). *Bereavement: studies of grief in adult life* (2nd edn). Taverstock Publications, New York. (The definitive reference book on bereavement.)

Rando, T. A. (1984). *Grief, dying, and death: clinical interventions for caregivers.* Research Press, Champaign, Illinois. (Valuable for those wishing to study in more depth.)

Worden, J. W. (1991). *Grief counselling and grief therapy.* (2nd edn). Tavistock Publications, London.

PASTORAL AND SPIRITUAL

Ainsworth-Smith, I. and Speck, P. (1983). *Letting go.* SPCK, London. (Spiritual and pastoral issues written by two hospital chaplains.)

Cassidy, S. (1988). *Sharing the darkness.* Darton, Longman, & Todd, London. (A sensitive, sympathetic book of value to professionals and lay carers.)

Fish, S. and Shelly, J. A. *Spiritual care: the nurse's role.* Intervarsity Press, Illinois. (A good text on spirituality and the nurse's response.)

Neuberger, J. (1987). *Caring for dying people of different faiths.* Lisa Sainsbury Foundation, Surrey/Austin Cornish Publishers. (An excellent booklet on the cultural and religious beliefs and practices of people of different faiths.)

Rumbold, B. D. *Helplessness and hope: pastoral care in terminal illness.* SCM Press, London. (Spiritual and pastoral care from the Christian perspective.)

Speck, P. (1978). *Loss and grief in medicine.* Ballière Tindall, London. (Spiritual and pastoral issues written by two hospital chaplains.)

FOR LITTLE CHILDREN

Snell, N. (1987). *Emma's cat dies*. Hamish Hamilton, London. (Ideal for the under-5's.)

FOR CHILDREN AND ADOLESCENTS

Krementz, J. (1983). *How it feels when a parent dies*. Victor Gollancz, London. (Most useful for younger readers.)

Mathias, B. and Speers, D. (1992). *A handbook on death and bereavement: helping children understand*. National Library for the Handicapped Child, Wokingham. (For children and adolescents.)

William, G. and Ross, J. (1983). *When people die*. Macdonald Publishers, Loanhead, Midlothian. (A book of simple, practical advice and support.)

St Christopher's Hospice Department of Social Work. (1991). *Your parent has died*.

FOR ADULTS

BACUP leaflets and booklets. This organization produces an excellent range of leaflets and books about different types of cancer and their treatment, written specifically for lay readers including the patients themselves. Obtainable from oncology departments or directly from BACUP, 121/123 Charterhouse Street, London EC1M 6AA.

Buckman, R. (1988). *I don't know what to say—how to help and support someone who is dying*. Macmillan, London. (A book of inestimable value to professionals and lay carers.)

Burton, L. (1974). *Care of the child facing death*. Routledge and Paul, London. (Guidance whether the child is dying or grieving another's death.)

Cassidy, S. (1988). *Sharing the darkness*. Darton, Longman, & Todd, London. (A sensitive, sympathetic book of value to professionals and lay carers.)

Doyle, D. (1994). *Caring for a dying relative*. Oxford University Press, Oxford. (A book intended to advise and encourage lay carers whether the dying relative is at home, in hospice, or in hospital.)

Kushner, H. S. (1981). *When bad things happen to good people*. Pan Books, London. (Written from a Christian perspective, helping grievers make sense of loss and grief.)

Lewis, M. (1992). *Tears and smiles*. Michael O'Mara Books Ltd, London. (A book about the 'Hospice Movement' by Martyn Lewis, the newscaster and author.)

Marshall, F. (1983). *Losing a parent*. Sheldon Press, SPCK, London. (Written for the adult coming to terms with loss.)

Rando, T. A. (1986). *Parental loss of a child*. Research Press, Champaign, Illinois. (About how it feels and how to cope when a young child dies.)

Richardson, J. (1979). *A death in the family*. Lion Publishing, Tring, Hertfordshire. (A helpful handbook on practical issues.)

Stedeford, A. (1994). *Facing death: patients, families, and professionals*. Second edition. Sobell Publications, Oxford. (A helpful book for professionals and caring relatives on the emotional problems and needs of all concerned, written by a psychiatrist experienced in palliative care.)

Index